Complications

A Surgeon's Notes on an Imperfect Science

Atul Gawande

Picador
A Metropolitan Book
Henry Holt and Company
New York

www.picadorusa.com

Picador® is a U.S. registered trademark and is used by Henry Holt and Company under license from Pan Books Limited.

For information on Picador Reading Group Guides, as well as ordering, please contact the Trade Marketing department at St. Martin's Press.
Phone: 1-800-221-7945 extension 763
Fax: 212-677-7456
E-mail: trademarketing@stmartins.com

Several of these pieces have appeared, in slightly different form, in *The New Yorker* and *Slate*.

Library of Congress Cataloging-in-Publication Data

Gawande, Atul.
   Complications : a young surgeon's notes on an imperfect science / Atul Gawande
      p. cm.
   Includes bibliographical references and index.
   ISBN 0-312-42170-2
   1. Surgeons—United States—Biography. 2. Surgery—Anecdotes.
I. Title.

RD27.35.G39 A3 2002
617'.092—dc21
[B]   2001055884

First published in the United States by Henry Holt and Company

20 19 18 17 16 15

FOR KATHLEEN

Contents

Complications

Author's Note

The stories here are true. In order to tell them while protecting people's confidentiality, however, I have needed to change the names of some patients, their families, and a few of my colleagues. In certain instances, I have also needed to change minor identifying details of individuals. Nonetheless, wherever such changes were made, I have indicated so in the body of the text.

Introduction

I was once on trauma duty when a young man about twenty years old was rolled in, shot in the buttock. His pulse, blood pressure, and breathing were all normal. A clinical assistant cut the clothes off him with heavy shears, and I looked him over from head to toe, trying to be systematic but quick about it. I found the entrance wound in his right cheek, a neat, red, half-inch hole. I could find no exit wound. No other injuries were evident.

He was alert and scared, more of us than of the bullet. "I'm fine," he insisted. "I'm *fine*." But on the rectal exam, my gloved finger came back coated with fresh blood. And when I threaded a urinary catheter into him, bright red flowed from his bladder, too.

The conclusion was obvious. The blood meant that the bullet had gone inside him, through both his rectum and his bladder, I told him. Major blood vessels, his kidney, other sections of bowel may have been hit as well. He needed surgery, I said, and we had to go now. He saw the look in my eyes, the nurses already packing him up to move, and he nodded, almost involuntarily, putting himself in our hands. Then the gurney wheels were whizzing, IV bags swinging, people holding doors open for us to pass through. In the operating room, the anesthesiologist put him under. We made a fast, deep slash down the middle of his abdomen, from his rib cage to his pubis. We grabbed retractors and pulled him open. And what we found inside was . . . nothing.

No blood. No hole in the bladder. No hole in the rectum. No bullet. We peeked under the drapes at the urine coming out of the catheter. It was normal now, clear yellow. It didn't have even a tinge of blood anymore. We had an X-ray machine brought into the room and got X rays of his pelvis, his abdomen, and also his chest. They showed no bullet anywhere. All of this was odd, to say the least. After almost an hour more of fruitless searching, however, there seemed nothing to do for him but sew him up. A couple days later we got yet another abdominal X ray. This one revealed a bullet lodged inside the right upper quadrant of his abdomen. We had no explanation for any of this—how a half-inch-long lead bullet had gotten from his buttock to his upper belly without injuring anything, why it hadn't appeared on the previous X rays, or where the blood we had seen had come from. Having already done more harm than the bullet had, however, we finally left it and the young man alone. We kept him in the hospital for a week. Except for our gash, he turned out fine.

Medicine is, I have found, a strange and in many ways disturbing business. The stakes are high, the liberties taken tremendous. We drug people, put needles and tubes into them, manipulate their chemistry, biology, and physics, lay them unconscious and open their bodies up to the world. We do so out of an abiding confidence in our know-how as a profession. What you find when you get in close, however—close enough to see the furrowed brows, the doubts and missteps, the failures as well as the successes—is how messy, uncertain, and also surprising medicine turns out to be.

The thing that still startles me is how fundamentally human an endeavor it is. Usually, when we think about medicine and its remarkable abilities, what comes to mind is the science and all it has given us to fight sickness and misery: the tests, the machines, the drugs, the procedures. And without question, these are at the center of virtually everything medicine achieves. But we rarely see how it all actually works. You have a cough that won't go away—and then? It's not science you call upon but a doctor. A doctor with good days and bad days. A doctor with a weird laugh and a bad haircut. A doctor with three other patients to see and, inevitably, gaps in what he knows and skills he's still trying to learn.

Recently, a boy was flown in by helicopter to one of the hospitals where I work as a resident. Lee Tran, as we can call him, was a small, spiky-haired kid barely out of elementary school. He had always been healthy. But for the previous week, his mother had noticed he had a dry, persistent cough and seemed less energetic than usual. For the last couple days he'd hardly eaten. She thought it was probably a flu. That evening, however, he came to her pale, tremulous, and wheezing, suddenly unable to catch his breath. At a local emergency room, the doctors gave him vaporized breathing treatments, thinking he was having an asthma attack. But then an X ray revealed an immense mass filling the middle of his chest. They got a CT scan for a more detailed picture. In stark black and white, it showed the mass to be a dense, almost football-size tumor enveloping the vessels to his heart, pushing the heart itself to one side, and compressing the airway to both lungs. The tumor had already completely crushed the passage to his right lung, and without air coming through, the lung had collapsed to a gray nubbin on the scan. A sea of fluid from the tumor occupied his right chest instead. Lee was living entirely off his left lung, and the tumor was pressing down on the airway to it, too. The community hospital he was in did not have the resources to deal with this. So the doctors there sent him to us. We had the specialists and high-tech equipment. But that didn't mean we were sure what to do.

By the time Lee arrived in our intensive care unit, his breathing was a buzzing, reedy stridor. You could hear it three beds away. The scientific literature is unequivocal about this situation: it is deadly dangerous. Just laying him down could cause the tumor to cut off the remainder of his airway. Giving him sedatives or anesthesia could do the same. Surgery to remove the tumor is impossible.

Chemotherapy, however, is known to shrink some of these tumors over the course of a few days. The question was how to buy the child time to find out. It wasn't clear he'd last the night.

We had two nurses, an anesthesiologist, a pediatric surgery junior fellow, and three residents at the bedside, myself included; the senior pediatric surgeon was on his cell phone, driving in from home; an oncologist was on page. One nurse propped Lee up on pillows to make sure he was as upright as he could be. The other put an oxygen mask on his face and hooked up monitors tracking his vital signs. The boy's eyes were wide and worried, and his breathing was about twice too fast. His family was still far away, having to travel by ground. But he remained sweetly brave, as children do more often than you'd expect.

My first instinct was that the anesthesiologist should put a stiff breathing tube into the boy's airway to fix it open before the tumor closed in. But the anesthesiologist thought this was nuts. She'd have to put the tube in without good sedation, with the kid sitting up, no less. And the tumor extended far along the airway. She wasn't convinced she could reach a tube past it easily enough.

The surgical fellow proposed another idea: if we put a catheter into the boy's right chest and drained off the fluid filling it, the tumor would tilt away from the left lung. On the phone, however, the senior surgeon was concerned that this could worsen matters. Once you have unsettled a boulder, can you honestly say which way it will roll? No one was thinking of any better options, however. So ultimately he said to go ahead.

I explained to Lee what we were going to do as simply as I could. I doubt he understood. That may have been just as well. After we'd gathered all the supplies we needed, two of us held Lee tight, and another injected a local anesthetic between his ribs, then made a slit with a knife and pushed a foot-and-a-half-long rubber catheter in. Bloody fluid poured out of the tube by the quart, and for a moment I was afraid we'd done something terrible. But as it turned out, we'd done more good than we could have hoped for. The tumor shifted rightward and somehow the airways to *both* lungs opened up. Instantly,

Lee's breathing became easier and quiet. After watching him a few minutes, so did ours.

Not until later did I wonder about our choice. It was little more than a guess about what to do—a stab in the dark, almost literally. We had no backup plan should disaster have occurred. And when I looked up reports of similar cases at the library afterward, I learned that other options did in fact exist. The safest thing, apparently, would have been to put him on a heart-lung bypass pump like the kind used during cardiac surgery, or at least to have one on standby. Talking with the others about it, though, I found that no one regretted a thing. Lee survived. That was what mattered. And his chemotherapy was now under way. Testing of the fluid showed the tumor to be a lymphoma. The oncologist told me that this gave Lee a better than 70 percent chance of total cure.

These are the moments in which medicine actually happens. And it is in these moments that this book takes place—the moments in which we can see and begin to think about the workings of things as they are. We look for medicine to be an orderly field of knowledge and procedure. But it is not. It is an imperfect science, an enterprise of constantly changing knowledge, uncertain information, fallible individuals, and at the same time lives on the line. There is science in what we do, yes, but also habit, intuition, and sometimes plain old guessing. The gap between what we know and what we aim for persists. And this gap complicates everything we do.

I am a surgical resident, very nearly at the end of my eight years of training in general surgery, and this book arises from the intensity of that experience. At other times I have been a laboratory scientist, a public health researcher, a student of philosophy and ethics, and a health policy adviser in government. I am also a son of two doctors, a husband, and a parent. I have attempted to bring all of these perspectives to bear on what I have written here. But more than anything, this book comes from what I have encountered and witnessed in the day-to-day caring of people. A resident has a distinctive vantage on medicine. You are an insider, seeing everything and a part of everything; yet at the same time you see it anew.

In some way, it may be in the nature of surgery itself to want to come to grips with the uncertainties and dilemmas of practical medicine. Surgery has become as high tech as medicine gets, but the best surgeons retain a deep recognition of the limitations of both science and human skill. Yet still they must act decisively.

The book's title, *Complications*, comes not just from the unexpected turns that can result in medicine but also, and more fundamentally, from my concern with the larger uncertainties and dilemmas that underlie what we do. This is the medicine that one cannot find explained in textbooks but that has puzzled me, sometimes troubled me, sometimes amazed me, as I've joined the profession's ranks. I have divided the book into three sections. The first examines the fallibility of doctors, asking, among other things, how mistakes happen, how a novice learns to wield a knife, what a good doctor is, how it is that one could go bad. The second focuses on mysteries and unknowns of medicine and the struggles with what to do about them; these are the stories of an architect with incapacitating back pain in whom no physical explanation could be found, a young woman with an awful nausea that would not go away, a television newscaster whose blushing became so inexplicably severe that she could no longer function in her job. The third and final section then centers on uncertainty itself. For what seems most vital and interesting is not how much we in medicine know but how much we don't—and how we might grapple with that ignorance more wisely.

Throughout I've sought to show not just the ideas but also the people in the middle of it all—the patients and doctors alike. In the end, it is practical, everyday medicine that most interests me—what happens when the simplicities of science come up against the complexities of individual lives. As pervasive as medicine has become in modern life, it remains mostly hidden and often misunderstood. We have taken it to be both more perfect than it is and less extraordinary than it can be.

Part I

Fallibility

Education of a Knife

The patient needed a central line. "Here's your chance," S., the chief resident, said. I had never done one before. "Get set up and then page me when you're ready to start."

It was my fourth week in surgical training. The pockets of my short white coat bulged with patient printouts, laminated cards with instructions for doing CPR and using the dictation system, two surgical handbooks, a stethoscope, wound-dressing supplies, meal tickets, a penlight, scissors, and about a buck in loose change. As I headed up the stairs to the patient's floor, I rattled.

This will be good, I tried to tell myself: my first real procedure. My patient—fiftyish, stout, taciturn—was recovering from abdominal surgery he'd had about a week before. His bowel function hadn't yet returned, leaving him unable to eat. I explained to him that he needed intravenous nutrition and that this required a "special line" that would go into his chest. I said that I would put the line in him while he was in his bed, and that it would involve my laying him out flat, numbing up a spot on his chest with local anesthetic, and then threading the line in. I did not say that the line was eight inches long and would go into his vena cava, the main blood vessel to his heart. Nor did I say how tricky the procedure would be. There were "slight risks" involved, I said, such as bleeding or lung collapse; in experienced hands, problems of this sort occur in fewer than one case in a hundred.

But, of course, mine were not experienced hands. And the disasters I knew about weighed on my mind: the woman who had died from massive bleeding when a resident lacerated her vena cava; the man who had had to have his chest opened because a resident lost hold of the wire inside the line which then floated down to the patient's heart; the man who had had a cardiac arrest when the procedure put him into ventricular fibrillation. But I said nothing of such things when I asked my patient's permission to do his line. And he said, "OK," I could go ahead.

I had seen S. do two central lines; one was the day before, and I'd attended to every step. I watched how she set out her instruments and laid down her patient and put a rolled towel between his shoulder blades to make his chest arch out. I watched how she swabbed his chest with antiseptic, injected lidocaine, which is a local anesthetic, and then, in full sterile garb, punctured his chest near his clavicle with a fat three-inch needle on a syringe. The patient didn't even flinch. S. told me how to avoid hitting the lung with the needle ("Go in at a steep angle; stay *right* under the clavicle"), and how to find the subclavian vein, a branch to the vena cava lying atop the lung near its apex ("Go in at a steep angle; stay *right* under the clavicle"). She pushed the needle in almost all the way. She drew back on the syringe. And she was in. You knew because the syringe filled with maroon blood. ("If it's bright red, you've hit an artery," she said. "That's not good.")

Once you have the tip of this needle poking in the vein, you have to widen the hole in the vein wall, fit the catheter in, and thread it in the right direction—down to the heart rather than up to the brain—all without tearing through vessels, lung, or anything else. To do this, S. explained, you start by getting a guidewire in place. She pulled the syringe off, leaving the needle in place. Blood flowed out. She picked up a two-foot-long twenty-gauge wire that looked like the steel D string of an electric guitar, and passed nearly its full length through the needle's bore, into the vein, and onward toward the vena cava. "Never force it in," she warned, "and never ever let go of it." A string of rapid heartbeats fired off on the cardiac monitor, and she quickly pulled the wire back an inch. It had poked into the heart, causing momentary fibrillation. "Guess we're in the right place," she said to me quietly. Then to the patient: "You're doing great. Only a couple minutes now." She pulled the needle out over the wire and replaced it with a bullet of thick, stiff plastic, which she pushed in tight to widen the vein opening. She then removed this dilator and threaded the central line—a spaghetti-thick, yellow, flexible plastic tube—over the wire until it was all the way in. Now she could remove the wire. She flushed the line with a heparin solution and sutured it to his chest. And that was it.

I had seen the procedure done. Now it was my turn to try. I set about gathering the supplies—a central-line kit, gloves, gown, cap, mask, lidocaine—and that alone took me forever. When I finally had the stuff together, I stopped outside my patient's door and just stood there staring, silently trying to recall the steps. They remained frustratingly hazy. But I couldn't put it off any longer. I had a page-long list of other things to get done: Mrs. A needed to be discharged; Mr. B needed an abdominal ultrasound arranged; Mrs. C needed her skin staples removed. . . . And every fifteen minutes or so I was getting paged with more tasks—Mr. X was nauseated and needed to be seen; Miss Y's family was here and needed "someone" to talk to them; Mr. Z needed a laxative. I took a deep breath, put on my best don't-worry-I-know-what-I'm-doing look, and went in to do the line.

I placed the supplies on a bedside table, untied the patient's gown behind his neck, and laid him down flat on the mattress, with his chest bare and his arms at his sides. I flipped on a fluorescent overhead light and raised his bed to my height. I paged S. to come. I put on my gown and gloves and, on a sterile tray, laid out the central line, guidewire, and other materials from the kit the way I remembered S. doing it. I drew up five cc's of lidocaine in a syringe, soaked two sponge-sticks in the yellow-brown Betadine antiseptic solution, and opened up the suture packaging. I was good to go.

S. arrived. "What's his platelet count?"

My stomach knotted. I hadn't checked. That was bad: too low and he could have a serious bleed from the procedure. She went to check a computer. The count was acceptable.

Chastened, I started swabbing his chest with the sponge-sticks. "Got the shoulder roll underneath him?" S. asked. Well, no. I had forgotten this, too. The patient gave me a look. S., saying nothing, got a towel, rolled it up, and slipped it under his back for me. I finished applying the antiseptic and then draped him so only his right upper chest was exposed. He squirmed a bit beneath the drapes. S. now inspected my tray. I girded myself.

"Where's the extra syringe for flushing the line when it's in?" Damn. She went out and got it.

I felt for landmarks on the patient's chest. *Here?* I asked with my eyes, not wanting to undermine my patient's confidence any further. She nodded. I numbed the spot with lidocaine. ("You'll feel a stick and a burn now, sir.") Next, I took the three-inch needle in hand and poked it through the skin. I advanced it slowly and uncertainly, a few millimeters at a time, afraid to plunge it into something bad. This is a big goddam needle, I kept thinking. I couldn't believe I was sticking it into someone's chest. I concentrated on maintaining a steep angle of entry, but kept spearing his clavicle instead of slipping beneath it.

"Ow!" he shouted.

"Sorry," I said. S. signaled with a kind of surfing hand gesture to go underneath the clavicle. This time it did. I drew back on the syringe. Nothing. She pointed deeper. I went in deeper. Nothing. I took the needle out, flushed out some bits of tissue clogging it, and tried again.

"*Ow!*"

Too superficial again. I found my way underneath the clavicle once more. I drew the syringe back. Still nothing. He's too obese, I thought to myself. S. slipped on gloves and a gown. "How about I have a look," she said. I handed her the needle and stepped aside. She plunged the needle in, drew back on the syringe, and, just like that, she was in. "We'll be done shortly," she told the patient. I felt utterly inept.

She let me continue with the next steps, which I bumbled through. I didn't realize how long and floppy the guidewire was until I pulled the coil out of its plastic sleeve, and, putting one end of it into the patient, I very nearly let the other touch his unsterile bed-sheet. I forgot about the dilating step until she reminded me. Then, when I put in the dilator, I didn't push quite hard enough, and it was really S. who pushed it all the way in. Finally we got the line in, flushed it, and sutured it in place.

Outside the room, S. said that I could be less tentative the next time, but that I shouldn't worry too much about how things had gone. "You'll get it," she said. "It just takes practice." I wasn't so sure. The procedure remained wholly mysterious to me. And I could not get over the idea of jabbing a needle so deeply and blindly into some-one's chest. I awaited the X ray afterward with trepidation. But it came back fine: I had not injured the lung and the line was in the right place.

Not everyone appreciates the attractions of surgery. When you are a medical student in the operating room for the first time, and you see the surgeon press the scalpel to someone's body and open it like fruit, you either shudder in horror or gape in awe. I gaped. It was not just the blood and guts that enthralled me. It was the idea that a mere person would have the confidence to wield that scalpel in the first place.

There is a saying about surgeons, meant as a reproof: "Some-times wrong; never in doubt." But this seemed to me their strength. Every day, surgeons are faced with uncertainties. Information is inadequate; the science is ambiguous; one's knowledge and abilities are never perfect. Even with the simplest operation, it cannot be taken for granted that a patient will come through better off—or even alive. Standing at the table my first time, I wondered how the surgeon knew that he would do this patient good, that all the steps would go as planned, that bleeding would be controlled and infection would not take hold and organs would not be injured. He didn't, of course. But still he cut.

Later, while still a student, I was allowed to make an incision myself. The surgeon drew a six-inch dotted line with a marking pen across a sleeping patient's abdomen and then, to my surprise, had the nurse hand me the knife. It was, I remember, still warm from the sterilizing autoclave. The surgeon had me stretch the skin taut with the thumb and forefinger of my free hand. He told me to make one smooth slice down to the fat. I put the belly of the blade to the skin and cut. The experience was odd and addictive, mixing exhilaration from the calculated violence of the act, anxiety about getting it right, and a righteous faith that it was somehow good for the person. There was also the slightly nauseating feeling of finding that it took more force than I'd realized. (Skin is thick and springy, and on my first pass I did not go nearly deep enough; I had to cut twice to get through.) The moment made me want to be a surgeon—not to be an amateur handed the knife for a brief moment, but someone with the confidence to proceed as if it were routine.

A resident, however, begins with none of this air of mastery—only a still overpowering instinct against doing anything like pressing a knife against flesh or jabbing a needle into someone's chest. On my first day as a surgical resident, I was assigned to the emergency room. Among my first patients was a skinny, dark-haired woman in her late twenties who hobbled in, teeth gritted, with a two-and-a-half-foot-long wooden chair-leg somehow nailed into the bottom of her foot. She explained that the leg had collapsed out from under a kitchen chair she had tried to sit upon and, leaping up to keep from falling, she inadvertently stomped her bare foot onto the three-inch screw sticking out of it. I tried very hard to look like someone who had not just got his medical diploma the week before. Instead, I was determined to be nonchalant, world-weary, the kind of guy who had seen this sort of thing a hundred times before. I inspected her foot and could see that the screw was imbedded in the bone at the base of her big toe. There was no bleeding, and, so far as I could feel, no fracture.

"Wow, that must hurt," I blurted out idiotically.

The obvious thing to do was give her a tetanus shot and pull out the screw. I ordered the tetanus shot, but I began to have doubts about pulling out the screw. Suppose she bled? Or suppose I fractured her foot? Or something worse? I excused myself and tracked down Dr. W, the senior surgeon on duty. I found him tending to a car-crash victim. The patient was a mess. People were shouting. Blood was all over the floor. It was not a good time to ask questions.

I ordered an X ray. I figured it would buy time and let me check my amateur impression that she didn't have a fracture. Sure enough, getting one took about an hour and it showed no fracture—just a common screw imbedded, the radiologist said, "in the head of the first metatarsal." I showed the patient the X ray. "You see, the screw's imbedded in the head of the first metatarsal," I said. And the plan? she wanted to know. Ah, yes, the plan.

I went to find Dr. W. He was still tied up with the crash victim, but I was able to interrupt to show him the X ray. He chuckled at the sight of it and asked me what I wanted to do. "Pull the screw out?" I ventured. "Yes," he said, by which he meant "Duh." He made sure I'd given a tetanus shot and then shooed me away.

Back in the room, I told her that I would pull the screw out, prepared for her to say something like "You?" Instead she said, "OK, Doctor," and it was time for me to get down to business. At first I had her sitting on the exam table, dangling her leg off the side. But that didn't look as if it would work. Eventually, I had her lie with her foot jutting off the end of the table, the board poking out into the air. With every move, her pain increased. I injected a local anesthetic where the screw went in and that helped a little. Now I grabbed her foot in one hand, the board in the other, and then for a moment I froze. Could I really do this? Should I really do this? Who was I to presume?

Finally, I just made myself do it. I gave her a one-two-three and pulled, too gingerly at first and then, forcing myself, hard. She groaned. The screw wasn't budging. I twisted, and abruptly it came free. There was no bleeding. I washed the wound out, as my textbooks said to for puncture wounds. She found she could walk, though the foot was sore. I warned her of the risks of infection and the signs to look for. Her gratitude was immense and flattering, like the lion's for the mouse—and that night I went home elated.

In surgery, as in anything else, skill and confidence are learned through experience—haltingly and humiliatingly. Like the tennis player and the oboist and the guy who fixes hard drives, we need practice to get good at what we do. There is one difference in medicine, though: it is people we practice upon.

My second try at placing a central line went no better than the first. The patient was in intensive care, mortally ill, on a ventilator, and needed the line so that powerful cardiac drugs could be delivered directly to her heart. She was also heavily sedated, and for this I was grateful. She'd be oblivious to my fumbling.

My preparation was better this time. I got the towel roll in place and the syringes of heparin on the tray. I checked her lab results, which were fine. I also made a point of draping more widely, so that if I flopped my guidewire around by mistake again, I could be sure it wouldn't hit anything unsterile.

For all that, the procedure was a bust. I stabbed the needle in too shallow and then too deep. Frustration overcame tentativeness and I tried one angle after another. Nothing worked. Then, for one brief moment, I got a flash of blood in the syringe, indicating I was in the vein. I anchored the needle with one hand and went to pull the syringe off with the other. But the syringe was jammed on too tightly, so that when I pulled it free I dislodged the needle from the vein.

The patient began bleeding into her chest wall. I applied pressure the best I could for a solid five minutes, but her chest still turned black and blue around the site. The hematoma made it impossible to put a line through there anymore. I wanted to give up. But she needed a line and the resident supervising me—a second-year this time—was determined that I succeed. After an X ray showed that I had not injured her lung, he had me try again on the other side with a whole new kit. I still missed, however, and before I turned the patient into a pincushion he took over. It took him several minutes and two or three sticks to find the vein himself and that made me feel better. Maybe she was an unusually tough case.

When I failed with a third patient a few days later, however, the doubts really set in. Again, it was stick, stick, stick, and nothing. I stepped aside. The resident watching me got it on the very next try.

Surgeons, as a group, adhere to a curious egalitarianism. They believe in practice, not talent. People often assume that you have to have great hands to become a surgeon, but it's not true. When I interviewed to get into surgery programs, no one made me sew or take a dexterity test or checked if my hands were steady. You do not even need all ten fingers to be accepted. To be sure, talent helps. Professors say every two or three years they'll see someone truly gifted come through a program—someone who picks up complex manual skills unusually quickly, sees the operative field as a whole, notices trouble before it happens. Nonetheless, attending surgeons say that what's most important to them is finding people who are conscientious, industrious, and boneheaded enough to stick at practicing this one difficult thing day and night for years on end. As one professor of surgery put it to me, given a choice between a Ph.D. who had painstakingly cloned a gene and a talented sculptor, he'd pick the Ph.D. every time. Sure, he said, he'd bet on the sculptor being more physically talented; but he'd bet on the Ph.D. being less "flaky." And in the end that matters more. Skill, surgeons believe, can be taught; tenacity cannot. It's an odd approach to recruitment, but it continues all the way up the ranks, even in top surgery departments. They take minions with no experience in surgery, spend years training them, and then take most of their faculty from these same home-grown ranks.

And it works. There have now been many studies of elite performers—international violinists, chess grand masters, professional ice-skaters, mathematicians, and so forth—and the biggest difference researchers find between them and lesser performers is the cumulative amount of deliberate practice they've had. Indeed, the most important talent may be the talent for practice itself. K. Anders Ericsson, a cognitive psychologist and expert on performance, notes that the most important way in which innate factors play a role may be in one's *willingness* to engage in sustained training. He's found, for example, that top performers dislike practicing just as much as others do. (That's why, for example, athletes and musicians usually quit practicing when they retire.) But more than others, they have the will to keep at it anyway.

I wasn't sure I did. What good was it, I wondered, to keep doing central lines when I wasn't coming close to getting them in? If I had a clear idea of what I was doing wrong, then maybe I'd have something to focus on. But I didn't. Everyone, of course, had suggestions. Go in with the bevel of the needle up. No, go in with the bevel down. Put a bend in the middle of the needle. No, curve the needle. For a while, I tried to avoid doing another line. Soon enough, however, a new case arose.

The circumstances were miserable. It was late in the day and I'd been up all the night before. The patient was morbidly obese, weighing more than three hundred pounds. He couldn't tolerate lying flat because the weight of his chest and abdomen made it hard for him to breathe. Yet he absolutely needed a central line. He had a badly infected wound and needed intravenous antibiotics, and no one could find veins in his arms for a peripheral IV. I had little hope of succeeding. But a resident does what he is told, and I was told to try the line.

I went to his room. He looked scared and said he didn't think he'd last more than a minute on his back. But he said he understood the situation and was willing to make his best effort. He and I decided that he'd be left sitting propped up in bed until the last possible minute. We'd see how far we got after that.

I went through my preparations: checking the labs, putting out the kit, placing the towel roll, and so on. I swabbed and draped his chest while he was still sitting up. S., the chief resident, was watching me this time, and when everything was ready I had her tip him back, an oxygen mask on his face. His flesh rolled up his chest like a wave. I couldn't find his clavicle with my fingertips to line up the right point of entry. And already he was looking short of breath, his face red. I gave S. a "Do you want to take over?" look. Keep going, she signaled. I made a rough guess as to where the right spot was, numbed it with lidocaine, then pushed the big needle in. For a second, I thought it wouldn't be long enough to reach through, but then I felt the tip slip underneath his clavicle. I pushed a little deeper and drew back on the syringe. Unbelievably, it filled with blood. *I was in.* I concentrated on anchoring the needle firmly in place, not moving it a millimeter as I pulled the syringe off and threaded the guidewire in. The wire fed in smoothly. He was struggling hard for air now. We sat him up and let him catch his breath. And then with one more lie-down, I got the entry dilated and slid the central line in. "Nice job," was all S. said, and then she left.

I still have no idea what I did differently that day. But from then on, my lines went in. Practice is funny that way. For days and days, you make out only the fragments of what to do. And then one day you've got the thing whole. Conscious learning becomes unconscious knowledge, and you cannot say precisely how.

I have now put in more than a hundred central lines. I am by no means infallible. Certainly, I have had my fair share of what we prefer to call "adverse events." I punctured a patient's lung, for example—the right lung of a surgeon from another hospital, no less—and, given the odds, I'm sure such things will happen again. I still have the occasional case that should go easily, but doesn't, no matter what I do. (We have a term for this. "How'd it go?" a colleague asks. "It was a total flog," I reply. I don't have to say anything more.)

But then there are the other times, when everything goes perfectly. You don't think. You don't concentrate. Every move unfolds effortlessly. You take the needle. You stick the chest. You feel the needle travel—a distinct glide through the fat, a slight catch in the dense muscle, then the subtle pop through the vein wall—and you're in. At such moments, it is more than easy; it is beautiful.

Surgical training is the recapitulation of this process—the floundering followed by fragments, followed by knowledge and occasionally a moment of elegance—over and over again, for ever harder tasks with ever greater risks. At first, you work on the basics: how to glove and gown, how to drape patients, how to hold the knife, how to tie a square knot in a length of silk suture (not to mention how to dictate, work the computers, order drugs). But then the tasks become more daunting: how to cut through skin, handle the electrocautery, open the breast, tie off a bleeding vessel, excise the tumor, close up the wound—a breast lumpectomy. By the end of six months, I had done lines, appendectomies, skin grafts, hernia repairs, and mastectomies. At the end of a year, I was doing limb amputations, lymph node biopsies, and hemorrhoidectomies. At the end of two years, I was doing tracheotomies, a few small-bowel operations, and laparoscopic gallbladder operations.

I am in my seventh year of training. Only now has a simple slice through skin begun to seem like nothing, the mere start of a case. When I'm inside, the struggle remains. These days, I'm trying to learn how to fix abdominal aortic aneurysms, remove pancreatic cancers, open blocked carotid arteries. I am, I have found, neither gifted nor maladroit. With practice and more practice, I get the hang of it.

We find it hard, in medicine, to talk about this with patients. The moral burden of practicing on people is always with us, but for the most part unspoken. Before each operation, I go over to the pre-operative holding area in my scrubs and introduce myself to the patient. I do it the same way every time. "Hello, I'm Dr. Gawande. I'm one of the surgical residents, and I'll be assisting your surgeon." That is pretty much all I say on the subject. I extend my hand and give a smile. I ask the patient if everything is going OK so far. We chat. I answer questions. Very occasionally, patients are taken aback. "No resident is doing my surgery," they say. I try to reassure. "Not to worry. I just assist," I say. "The attending surgeon is always in charge."

None of this is exactly a lie. The attending *is* in charge, and a resident knows better than to forget that. Consider the operation I did recently to remove a seventy-five-year-old woman's colon cancer. The attending stood across from me from the start. And it was he, not I, who decided where to cut, how to isolate the cancer, how much colon to take.

Yet to say I just assisted remains a kind of subterfuge. I wasn't merely an extra pair of hands, after all. Otherwise, why did I hold the knife? Why did I stand on the operator's side of the table? Why was it raised to my six-feet-plus height? I was there to help, yes, but I was there to practice, too. This was clear when it came time to reconnect the colon. There are two ways of putting the ends together—by hand-sewing them or stapling them. Stapling is swifter and easier, but the attending suggested I hand-sew the ends—not because it was better for the patient but because I had done it few times before. When it's performed correctly, the results are similar, but he needed to watch me like a hawk. My stitching was slow and imprecise. At one point, he caught me leaving the stitches too far apart and made me go back and put extras in between so the connection would not leak. At another point, he found I wasn't taking deep enough bites of tissue with the needle to insure a strong closure. "Turn your wrist more," he told me. "Like this?" I asked. "Uh, sort of," he said. I was learning.

In medicine, we have long faced a conflict between the imperative to give patients the best possible care and the need to provide novices with experience. Residencies attempt to mitigate potential harm through supervision and graduated responsibility. And there is reason to think patients actually benefit from teaching. Studies generally find teaching hospitals have better outcomes than non-teaching hospitals. Residents may be amateurs, but having them around checking on patients, asking questions, and keeping faculty on their toes seems to help. But there is still no getting around those first few unsteady times a young physician tries to put in a central line, remove a breast cancer, or sew together two segments of colon. No matter how many protections we put in place, on average these cases go less well with the novice than with someone experienced.

We have no illusions about this. When an attending physician brings a sick family member in for surgery, people at the hospital think hard about how much to let trainees participate. Even when the attending insists that they participate as usual, a resident scrubbing in knows that it will be far from a teaching case. And if a central line must be put in, a first-timer is certainly not going to do it. Conversely, the ward services and clinics where residents have the most responsibility are populated by the poor, the uninsured, the drunk, and the demented. Residents have few opportunities nowadays to operate independently, without the attending docs scrubbed in, but when we do—as we must before graduating and going out to operate on our own—it is generally on these, the humblest of patients.

This is the uncomfortable truth about teaching. By traditional ethics and public insistence (not to mention court rulings), a patient's right to the best care possible must trump the objective of training novices. We want perfection without practice. Yet everyone is harmed if no one is trained for the future. So learning is hidden, behind drapes and anesthesia and the elisions of language. Nor does the dilemma apply just to residents, physicians in training. In fact, the process of learning turns out to extend longer than most people know.

My sister and I grew up in the small town of Athens, Ohio, where our parents are both doctors. Long ago my mother chose to practice pediatrics part-time, only three half-days a week, and she was able to because my father's urology practice became so busy and successful. He has now been at it for more than twenty-five years, and his office is cluttered with the evidence of it: an overflowing wall of patient files, gifts from people displayed everywhere (books, paintings, ceramics with biblical sayings, hand-painted paperweights, blown glass, and carved boxes, as well as a figurine of a boy who pees on you when you pull down his pants). In an acrylic case behind his oak desk there are a few dozen of the thousands of kidney stones he has removed from these patients.

Only now, as I get glimpses of the end of my training, have I begun to think hard about my father's success. For most of residency, I thought of surgery as a more or less fixed body of knowledge and skill which is acquired in training and perfected in practice. There was, as I envisioned it, a smooth, upward-sloping arc of proficiency at some rarefied set of tasks (for me, taking out gallbladders, colon cancers, bullets, and appendices; for him, taking out kidney stones, testicular cancers, and swollen prostates). The arc would peak at, say, ten or fifteen years, plateau for a long time, and perhaps tail off a little in the final five years before retirement. The reality, however, turns out to be far messier. You do get good at certain things, my father tells me, but no sooner than you do, you find what you know is outmoded. New technologies and operations emerge to supplant the old, and the learning curve starts all over again. "Three-quarters of what I do today I never learned in residency," he says. On his own, fifty miles from his nearest colleague—let alone a doctor who could tell him anything like "You need to turn your wrist more when you do that"—he has had to learn to put in penile prostheses, to perform microsurgery, to reverse vasectomies, to do nerve-sparing prostatec-tomies, to implant artificial urinary sphincters. He's had to learn to use shock-wave lithotripters, electrohydraulic lithotripters, and laser lithotripters (all instruments for breaking up kidney stones); to deploy Double J ureteral stents and Silicone Figure Four Coil stents and Retro-Inject Multi-Length stents (don't even ask); to maneuver fiber-optic ureteroscopes. All these technologies and techniques were introduced since he finished training. Some of the procedures built on previous skills. Many did not.

This is, in fact, the experience all surgeons have. The pace of medical innovation has been unceasing, and surgeons have no choice but to give the new new thing a try. To fail to adopt new tech-niques would mean denying patients meaningful medical advances. Yet the perils of the learning curve are inescapable—no less in prac-tice than in residency.

For the established surgeon, inevitably, the opportunities for learning are far less structured than for a resident. When an impor-tant new device or procedure comes along, as they do every year, sur-geons start out by taking a course about it—typically a day or two of lectures by some surgical grandees with a few film clips and step-by-step handouts. We take a video home to watch. Perhaps we pay a visit to observe a colleague perform the operation—my father often goes up to Ohio State or the Cleveland Clinic for this. But there's not much by way of hands-on training. Unlike a resident, a visitor cannot scrub in on cases, and opportunities to practice on animals or cadav-ers are few and far between. (Britain, being Britain, actually bans surgeons from practicing on animals.) When the pulsed-dye laser came out, the manufacturer set up a lab in Columbus where urolo-gists from the area could gain experience. But when my father went, the main experience provided was destroying kidney stones in test tubes filled with a urinelike liquid and trying to penetrate the shell of an egg without hitting the membrane underneath. My surgery department recently purchased a robotic surgery device—a stagger-ingly sophisticated nine-hundred-and-eighty-thousand-dollar robot, with three arms, two wrists, and a camera, all millimeters in diameter, which, controlled from a console, allows a surgeon to do almost any operation with absolutely no hand tremor and with only tiny incisions. A team of two surgeons and two nurses flew out to the manufacturer's headquarters in San Jose for a full day of training on the machine. And they did get to practice on a pig and on a human cadaver. (The company apparently buys the cadavers from the city of San Francisco.) But even this, which is far more practice than one usually gets, was hardly thorough training. They learned enough to grasp the principles for operating the robot, to start getting a feel for using it, and to understand how to plan an operation. That was about it. Sooner or later, one just has to go home and give the thing a try.

Patients do eventually benefit—often enormously—but the first few patients may not and may even be harmed. Consider the experience reported by the pediatric-surgery unit of the renowned Great Ormond Street Hospital in London, as detailed in the *British Medical Journal* in the spring of 2000. The doctors described their results in operating on three hundred and twenty-five consecutive babies with a severe heart defect, known as transposition of the great arteries, over a period (from 1978 to 1998) when its surgeons changed from doing one operation for the condition to another. Such children are born with their heart's outflow vessels transposed: the aorta emerges from the right side of the heart instead of the left and the artery to the lungs emerges from the left instead of the right. As a result, blood coming in is pumped right back out to the body instead of first to the lungs, where it can be oxygenated. This is unsurvivable. The babies died blue, fatigued, never knowing what it was to get enough breath. For years, switching the vessels to their proper positions wasn't technically feasible. Instead, surgeons did something known as the Senning procedure: they created a passage inside the heart to let blood from the lungs cross backward to the right heart. The Senning procedure allowed children to live into adulthood. The weaker right heart, however, cannot sustain the body's entire blood flow as long as the left. Eventually, these patients' hearts failed, and although most made it to adulthood, few lived to old age. Then, by the 1980s, a series of technological advancements made it possible to do a switch operation safely. It rapidly became the favored procedure. In 1986, the Great Ormond Street surgeons made the changeover, and their report shows that it was unquestionably a change for the better. The annual death rate after a successful switch procedure was less than a quarter that after the Senning, resulting in a life expectancy of sixty-three years instead of forty-seven. But the price of learning to do it was appalling. In their first seventy switch operations, the doctors had a 25 percent surgical death rate, compared with just 6 percent with the Senning procedure. (Eighteen babies died, more than twice the number of the entire Senning era.) Only with time did they master it: in their next hundred switch operations, just five babies died.

As patients, we want both expertise and progress. What nobody wants to face is that these are contradictory desires. In the words of one British public report, "There should be no learning curve as far as patient safety is concerned." But that is entirely wishful thinking.

Recently, a group of Harvard Business School researchers who have made a specialty of studying learning curves in industry—in making semiconductors, building airplanes, and such—decided to examine learning curves among surgeons. They followed eighteen cardiac surgeons and their teams as they took on the new technique of minimally invasive cardiac surgery. This study, I was surprised to discover, is the first of its kind. Learning is ubiquitous in medicine, and yet no one had ever compared how well different clinicians actually do it.

The new heart operation—involving a small incision between ribs instead of a chest split open down the middle—proved substantially more difficult than the conventional one. Because the incision is too small to admit the usual tubes and clamps for rerouting blood to the heart-bypass machine, surgeons had to learn a trickier method, which involved balloons and catheters placed through groin vessels.

They had to learn how to operate in a much reduced space. And the nurses, anesthesiologists, and perfusionists all had new roles to master, too. Everyone had new tasks, new instruments, new ways that things could go wrong, and new ways to fix them. As you'd expect, everyone was found to experience a substantial learning curve. Whereas a fully proficient team takes three to six hours for such operations, these teams took an average of three times longer for their early cases. The researchers could not track rates of morbidity in detail, but it would be foolish to imagine that these rates were not affected.

What's more interesting is that researchers found striking disparities in the speed with which different teams learned. All teams received the same three-day training session and came from highly respected institutions with experience in adopting innovations. Yet, in the course of fifty cases, some teams managed to halve their operating time while others failed to improve at all. Practice, it turned out, did not necessarily make perfect. Whether it did, the researchers found, depended on *how* the surgeons and their teams practiced.

Richard Bohmer, the one physician among the Harvard researchers, made several visits to observe one of the quickest-learning teams and one of the slowest, and he was startled by the contrast. The surgeon on the fast-learning team was actually quite inexperienced compared with the one on the slow-learning team—he was only a couple of years out of training. But he made sure to pick team members with whom he had worked well before and to keep them together through the first fifteen cases before allowing any new members. He had the team go through a dry run before the first case, then deliberately scheduled six operations in the first week, so little would be forgotten in between. He convened the team before each case to discuss it in detail and afterward to debrief. He made sure results were tracked carefully. And as a person, Bohmer noticed, the surgeon was not the stereotypical Napoleon with a knife. Unbidden, he told Bohmer, "The surgeon needs to be willing to allow himself to become a partner [with the rest of the team] so he can accept input." It sounded perhaps a little clichéd; but then again, whatever he was doing worked. At the other hospital, the surgeon chose his operating team almost randomly and did not keep it together. In his first seven cases, the team had different members every time, which is to say that it was no team at all. And he had no pre-briefings, no debriefings, no tracking of ongoing results.

The Harvard Business School study offered some hopeful news. We can do things that have a dramatic effect on the learning curve—like being more deliberate about how we train, and about tracking progress, whether with students and residents or senior surgeons and nurses. But the study's other findings are less reassuring. No matter how accomplished, surgeons trying something new got worse before they got better, and the learning curve proved longer, and affected by a far more complicated range of factors, than anyone had realized. It's all stark confirmation that you can't train novices without compromising patient care.

This, I suspect, is the reason for the physician's dodge: the "I just assist" rap; the "We have a new procedure for this that you are perfect for" speech; the "You need a central line" without the "I am still learning how to do this." Sometimes we do feel obliged to admit when we're doing something for the first time, but even then we tend to quote the published success rates—which are virtually always from experienced surgeons. Do we ever tell patients that because we are still new at something, their risks will inevitably be higher, and that they'd likely do better with others who are more experienced? Do we ever say that we need them to agree to it anyway? I've never seen it. Given the stakes, who in their right mind would agree to be practiced upon?

Many dispute this presumption. "Look, most people understand what it is to be a doctor," a health policy expert insisted, when I visited his office not long ago. "We have to stop lying to our patients. Can people take on chances for societal benefit?" He paused and then answered his question. "Yes," he said firmly.

It would certainly be a graceful and happy solution. We'd ask patients—honestly, openly—and then they'd say yes. Hard to imagine, though. I noticed on the expert's desk a picture of his child, born just a few months before, and a completely unfair question popped into my mind. "So did you let the resident deliver?" I asked.

There was silence for a moment. "No," he admitted. "We didn't even allow residents in the room."

One reason I doubt that we could sustain a system of medical training that depended on people saying "Yes, you can practice upon me" is that I myself have said no. One Sunday morning, when my eldest child, Walker, was eleven days old, he suddenly went into congestive heart failure from what proved to be a severe cardiac defect. His aorta was not transposed, but a long segment of it had failed to grow at all. My wife and I were beside ourselves with fear—his kidneys and liver began failing, too—but he made it to surgery, the repair was a success, and although his recovery was erratic, after two and a half weeks he was ready to come home.

We were by no means home free, however. He was born a healthy six pounds plus but now, at a month of age, weighed only five, and would need strict monitoring to insure that he gained weight. He was on two cardiac medications from which he would have to be weaned. And in the longer term, the doctors warned us, his repair would eventually prove inadequate. As Walker grew, his aorta would require either dilation with a balloon or wholesale replacement in surgery. Precisely when and how many such procedures would be necessary over the years they could not say. A pediatric cardiologist would have to follow him closely and decide.

Nearing discharge, we had not chosen who that cardiologist would be. In the hospital, Walker had been cared for by a full team of cardiologists, ranging from fellows in specialty training to attendings who had practiced for decades. The day before discharge, one of the young fellows approached me, offering his card and a suggested appointment time to bring Walker to see him. Of those on the team, he was the one who had put in the most time caring for Walker. He was the one who saw Walker when we brought him in inexplicably short of breath, the one who made the diagnosis, who got Walker the drugs that stabilized him, who coordinated with the surgeons, and who came to see us each day to answer our questions. Moreover, I knew fellows always got their patients this way. Most families don't know the subtle gradations among players, and after a team has saved their child's life, they take whatever appointment they're handed.

But I knew the differences. "I'm afraid we're thinking of seeing Dr. Newburger," I said. She was the hospital's associate cardiologist-in-chief, and a published expert on conditions like Walker's. The young physician looked crestfallen. It was nothing against him, I said. She just had more experience, that was all.

"You know, there is always an attending backing me up," he said. I shook my head.

I know this was not fair. My son had an unusual problem. The fellow needed the experience. Of all people, I, a resident, should have understood. But I was not torn about the decision. This was *my child*. Given a choice, I will always choose the best care I can for him. How can anybody be expected to do otherwise? Certainly, the future of medicine should not rely on it.

In a sense, then, the physician's dodge is inevitable. Learning must be stolen, taken as a kind of bodily eminent domain. And it was, during Walker's stay—on many occasions, now that I think back on it. A resident intubated him. A surgical trainee scrubbed in for his operation. The cardiology fellow put in one of his central lines. None of them asked me if they could. If offered the option to have someone more experienced, I certainly would have taken it. But that was simply how the system worked—no such choices were offered—and so I went along. What else could I do?

The advantage of this coldhearted machinery is not merely that it gets the learning done. If learning is necessary but causes harm, then above all it ought to apply to everyone alike. Given a choice, people wriggle out, and those choices are not offered equally. They belong to the connected and the knowledgeable, to insiders over outsiders, to the doctor's child but not the truck driver's. If choice cannot go to everyone, maybe it is better when it is not allowed at all.

It is 2 P.M. I am in the intensive care unit. A nurse tells me Mr. G's central line has clotted off. Mr. G has been with us for more than a month now. He is in his late sixties, from South Boston, emaciated, exhausted, holding on by a thread—or a line, to be precise. He has several holes in his small bowel that surgery has failed to close, and the bilious contents leak out onto his skin through two small reddened openings in the concavity of his abdomen. His only chance is to be fed by vein and wait for these fistulae to heal. He needs a new central line.

I could do it, I suppose. I am the experienced one now. But experience brings a new role: I am expected to teach the procedure instead. "See one, do one, teach one," the saying goes, and it is only half in jest.

There is a junior resident on the service. She has done only one or two lines before. I tell her about Mr. G. I ask her if she is free to do a new line. She misinterprets this as a question. She says she still has patients to see and a case coming up later. Could I do the line? I tell her no. She is unable to hide a grimace. She is burdened, as I was burdened, and perhaps frightened, as I was frightened.

She begins to focus when I make her talk through the steps— a kind of dry run, I figure. She hits nearly all the steps, but crucially forgets about checking the labs and about Mr. G's nasty allergy to heparin, which is in the flush for the line. I make sure she registers this, then tell her to get set up and page me.

I am still adjusting to this role. It is painful enough taking responsibility for one's own failures. Being handmaiden to another's is something else entirely. It occurs to me that I could have broken open a kit and had her do an actual dry run. Then again, maybe I can't. The kits must be a couple of hundred dollars each. I'll have to find out for next time.

Half an hour later, I get the page. The patient is draped. The resident is in her gown and gloves. She tells me she has saline to flush the line with and that his labs are fine.

"Have you got the towel roll?" I ask.

She forgot the towel roll. I roll up a towel and slip it beneath Mr. G's back. I look into his face and ask him if he's all right. He nods. I see no fear. After all he's been through, there is only resignation.

The junior resident picks out a spot for the stick. The patient is so hauntingly thin. I see every rib and fear she will puncture his lung. She injects the numbing medication. Then she puts the big needle in, and the angle looks all wrong. I motion for her to reposition. This only makes her more uncertain. She pushes in deeper and I know she does not have it. She draws back on the syringe: no blood. She takes out the needle and tries again. And again, the angle looks wrong. This time Mr. G feels the jab and jerks up in pain. I hold his arm. She gives him more numbing medication. It is all I can do not to take over. But she cannot learn without doing, I tell myself. I decide to let her have one more try.

printout. The theory behind an EKG is that in a heart attack a portion of the muscle dies, causing the electrical impulses to change course when they travel around the dead tissue. As a result, the waves on the printout change, too. Sometimes those changes are obvious; more often they are subtle—or, in medical argot, "nonspecific."

To medical students, EKGs seem unmanageably complex at first. Typically, an EKG uses twelve leads, and each one produces a different-looking tracing on the printout. Yet students are taught to discern in these tracings a dozen or more features, each of which is given an alphabetical label: for instance, there's the downstroke at the start of a beat (the Q wave), the upstroke at the peak of heart contraction (the R wave), the subsequent downstroke (the S wave), and the rounded wave right after the beat (the T wave). Sometimes small changes here and there add up to a heart attack; sometimes they don't. When I was a medical student, I first learned to decode the EKG as if it were a complex calculation. My classmates and I would carry laminated cards in our white-lab-coat pockets with a list of arcane instructions: calculate the heart rate and the axis of electrical flow, check for a rhythm disturbance, then check for an ST-segment elevation greater than one millimeter in leads V_1 to V_4, or for poor R-wave progression (signifying one type of heart attack), and so on.

With practice, it gets easier to manage all this information, just as putting a line in gets easier. The learning curve operates in matters of diagnosis no less than technique. An experienced cardiologist can sometimes make out a heart attack at a glance, the way a child can recognize his mother across a room. But at bottom the test remains stubbornly opaque. Studies have shown that between 2 and 8 percent of patients with heart attacks who are seen in emergency rooms are mistakenly discharged, and a quarter of these people die or suffer a complete cardiac arrest. Even if such patients aren't mistakenly sent home, crucial treatment may be delayed when an EKG is misread. Human judgment, even expert human judgment, falls well short of certainty. The rationale for trying to teach a computer to read an EKG, therefore, is fairly compelling. If the result should prove to be even a slight improvement on human performance, thousands of lives could be saved each year.

The first suggestion that a computer could do better came in 1990, in an influential article published by William Baxt, then an emergency physician at the University of California at San Diego. Baxt described how an "artificial neural network"—a kind of computer architecture—could make sophisticated clinical decisions. Such expert systems learn from experience much as humans do: by incorporating feedback from each success and each failure to improve their guesswork. In a later study, Baxt showed that a computer could handily outperform a group of doctors in diagnosing heart attacks among patients with chest pain. But two-thirds of the physicians in his study were inexperienced residents, whom you'd expect to have difficulties with EKGs. Could a computer outperform an experienced specialist?

This question was what the Swedish study was trying to answer. The study was led by Lars Edenbrandt, a medical colleague of Ohlin's and an expert in artificial intelligence. Edenbrandt spent five years perfecting his system, first in Scotland and then in Sweden. He fed his computer EKGs from more than ten thousand patients, telling it which ones represented heart attacks and which ones did not, until the machine grew expert at reading even the most equivocal of EKGs. Then he approached Ohlin, one of the top cardiologists in Sweden and a man who ordinarily read as many as ten thousand EKGs a year. Edenbrandt selected two thousand two hundred and forty EKGs from the hospital files to test both of them on, of which exactly half, eleven hundred and twenty, were confirmed to show heart attacks. With little fanfare, the results were published in the fall of 1997. Ohlin correctly picked up six hundred and twenty. The computer picked up seven hundred and thirty-eight. Machine beat man by 20 percent.

Western medicine is dominated by a single imperative—the quest for machinelike perfection in the delivery of care. From the first day of medical training, it is clear that errors are unacceptable.

Taking time to bond with patients is fine, but every X ray must be tracked down and every drug dose must be exactly right. No allergy or previous medical problem can be forgotten, no diagnosis missed. In the operating room, no movement, no time, no drop of blood can be wasted.

The keys to this kind of perfection are routinization and repetition: survival rates after heart surgery, vascular surgery, and other operations are directly related to the number of procedures the surgeon has performed. Twenty-five years ago, general surgeons performed hysterectomies, removed lung cancers, and bypassed hardened leg arteries. Today, each condition has its specialists, who perform one narrow set of procedures over and over again. When I'm in the operating room, the highest praise I can receive from my fellow surgeons is "You're a machine, Gawande." And the use of "machine" is more than casual: human beings, under some circumstances, really can act like machines.

Consider a relatively simple surgical procedure, a hernia repair, which I learned to do as a first-year surgical resident. A hernia is a weakening of the abdominal wall, usually in the groin, that allows the abdomen's contents to bulge through. In most hospitals, fixing it—pushing the bulge back in and repairing the abdominal wall—takes about ninety minutes and might cost upward of four thousand dollars. In anywhere from 10 to 15 percent of the cases, the operation eventually fails and the hernia returns. There is, however, a small medical center outside Toronto, known as the Shouldice Hospital, where none of these statistics apply. At Shouldice, hernia operations often take from thirty to forty-five minutes. Their recurrence rate is an astonishing 1 percent. And the cost of an operation is about half of what it is elsewhere. There's probably no better place in the world to get a hernia repaired.

What's the secret of that clinic's success? The short answer is that the dozen surgeons at Shouldice do hernia operations and nothing else. Each surgeon repairs between six hundred and eight hundred hernias a year—more than most general surgeons do in a lifetime. In this particular field, Shouldice's staff is better trained and has more experience than anyone else. But there's another way to formulate the reason for its success, which is that all the repetition changes the way they think. As Lucian Leape, a Harvard pediatric surgeon who has made a study of medical error, explains, "a defining trait of experts is that they move more and more problem-solving into an automatic mode." With repetition, a lot of mental functioning becomes automatic and effortless, as when you drive a car to work. Novel situations, however, usually require conscious thought and "workaround" solutions, which are slower to develop, more difficult to execute, and more prone to error. A surgeon for whom most situations have automatic solutions has a significant advantage. If the Swedish EKG study argues that there are situations in which machines should replace physicians, the Shouldice example suggests that physicians should be trained to act more like machines.

One chilly Monday morning, I put on a green cotton scrub top and pants, a disposable mask, and a paper cap, and wandered among cases in the Shouldice Hospital's five operating rooms. To describe one case is to describe them all: I watched three surgeons operate on six patients, and none deviated even a step from their standard protocol.

In a tiled, boxlike operating room, I peered over the shoulder of Richard Sang, a fifty-one-year-old surgeon with a dry wit and a youthful appearance. Though we chatted during the entire operation, Dr. Sang performed each step without pause, almost absently, with the assistant knowing precisely which tissues to retract, and the nurse handing over exactly the right instruments; instructions were completely unnecessary. The patient, a pleasant, surprisingly composed man of about thirty-five, who occasionally piped up from under the drapes to ask how things were going, lay on the table with his lower abdomen exposed and painted yellow with a bactericidal iodine solution. A plum-size bulge was visible to the left side of the hard bone of the pubis. Dr. Sang injected the skin with a local anesthetic in a diagonal line from the top of the man's left hip to the pubis, along the crease of the groin. With a No. 10 blade, he made a four-inch slash along this line in a single downstroke, revealing yellow, glistening fat below. The assistant laid a cloth along each side of the wound to absorb the mild bleeding, and pulled it open.

Sang swiftly cut down through the outer muscle layer of the abdominal wall, exposing the spermatic cord, a half-inch cable of blood and spermatic vessels. The patient's bulge, we could now see, came through a weakness in the muscle wall beneath the cord, which is a common site. Sang slowed down for a moment, checking meticulously for another hernia, along the area where the cord came through the inner abdominal wall. Sure enough, he found a small, second hernia there—one that, if it had been missed, would almost certainly have caused a recurrence. He then sliced open the remaining muscle layers beneath the cord, so that the abdominal wall was completely open, and pushed the bulging abdominal contents back inside. If you have a tear in a couch cushion with stuffing coming through it, you can put a patch on the cushion or you can sew it back together. At my hospital, we usually push the hernia back in, place a piece of sturdy plasticlike mesh on top, and sew it to the surrounding tissue. It provides a reliable reinforcement, and the technique is easy to perform. But Sang, like the other Shouldice surgeons I asked, scoffed at the idea: they viewed the mesh as a hazard for infection (since it's a foreign body), expensive (since the mesh can cost hundreds of dollars), and unnecessary (since they get enviable results without it).

As Sang and I talked about such alternatives, he sewed the wall back together in three separate muscle layers, using fine wire, making sure that the edge of each layer overlapped like a double-breasted suit. After Sang closed the patient's skin with small clips and removed the drapes, the patient swung his legs over the edge of the table, stood up, and walked out of the room. The procedure had taken just half an hour.

Many surgeons elsewhere use Shouldice's distinctive repair method but obtain ordinary rates of recurrence. It's not the technique that makes Shouldice great. The doctors at Shouldice deliver hernia repairs the way Intel makes chips: they like to call themselves a "focused factory." Even the hospital building is specially designed for hernia patients. Their rooms have no phones or televisions, and their meals are served in a downstairs dining hall; as a result, the patients have no choice but to get up and walk around, thereby preventing problems associated with inactivity, such as pneumonia or leg clots.

After Sang left the patient with a nurse, he found the next patient and walked him straight back into the same operating room. Hardly three minutes had passed, but the room was already clean. Fresh sheets and new instruments were already laid out. And so the next case began. I asked Byrnes Shouldice, a son of the clinic's founder and a hernia surgeon himself, whether he ever got bored doing hernias all day long. "No," he said in a Spock-like voice. "Perfection is the excitement."

Paradoxically, this kind of superspecialization raises the question of whether the best medical care requires fully trained doctors. None of the three surgeons I watched operate at the Shouldice Hospital would even have been in a position to conduct their own procedures in a typical American hospital, for none had completed general surgery training. Sang was a former family physician; Byrnes Shouldice had come straight from medical school; and the surgeon-in-chief was an obstetrician. Yet after apprenticing for a year or so they were the best hernia surgeons in the world. If you're going to do nothing but fix hernias or perform colonoscopies, do you really need the complete specialists' training (four years of medical school, five or more years of residency) in order to excel? Depending on the area of specialization, do you—and this is the question posed by the Swedish EKG study—even have to be human?

Although the medical establishment has begun to recognize that automation like the Shouldice's may be able to produce better results in medical treatment, many doctors are not fully convinced. And they have been particularly reluctant to apply the same insight to the area of medical diagnosis. Most physicians believe that diagnosis can't be reduced to a set of generalizations—to a "cookbook," as some say. Instead, they argue, it must take account of the idiosyncrasies of individual patients.

This only stands to reason, doesn't it? When I am the surgical consultant in the emergency department, I'm often asked to assess whether a patient with abdominal pain has appendicitis. I listen closely to his story and consider a multitude of factors: how his abdomen feels to me, the pain's quality and location, his temperature, his appetite, the laboratory results. But I don't plug it all into a formula and calculate the result. I use my clinical judgment—my intuition—to decide whether he should undergo surgery, be kept in the hospital for observation, or be sent home. We've all heard about individuals who defy the statistics—the hardened criminal who goes straight, the terminal cancer patient who miraculously recovers. In psychology, there's something called the broken-leg problem. A statistical formula may be highly successful in predicting whether or not a person will go to a movie in the next week. But someone who knows that this person is laid up with a broken leg will beat the formula. No formula can take into account the infinite range of such exceptional events. That's why doctors are convinced that they'd better stick with their well-honed instincts when they're making a diagnosis.

One weekend on duty, I saw a thirty-nine-year-old woman with pain in the right-lower abdomen who did not fit the pattern for appendicitis. She said that she was fairly comfortable and she had no fever or nausea. Indeed, she was hungry, and she did not jump when I pressed on her abdomen. Her test results were largely equivocal. But I still recommended appendectomy to the attending surgeon. Her white blood cell count was high, suggesting infection, and, moreover, she just looked sick to me. Sick patients can have a certain unmistakable appearance you come to recognize after a while in residency. You may not know exactly what is going on, but you're sure it's something worrisome. The attending physician accepted my diagnosis, operated, and found appendicitis.

Not long after, I had a sixty-five-year-old patient with almost precisely the same story. The lab findings were the same; I also got an abdominal scan, but it was inconclusive. Here, too, the patient didn't fit the pattern for appendicitis; here, too, he just looked to me as if he had it. In surgery, however, the appendix turned out to be normal. He had diverticulitis, a colon infection that usually doesn't require an operation.

Is the second case more typical than the first? How often does my intuition lead me astray? The radical implication of the Swedish study is that the individualized, intuitive approach that lies at the center of modern medicine is flawed—it causes more mistakes than it prevents. There's ample support for this conclusion from studies outside medicine. Over the past four decades, cognitive psychologists have shown repeatedly that a blind algorithmic approach usually trumps human judgment in making predictions and diagnoses. The psychologist Paul Meehl, in his classic 1954 treatise, *Clinical Versus Statistical Prediction*, described a study of Illinois parolees that compared estimates given by prison psychiatrists that a convict would violate parole with estimates derived from a rudimentary formula that weighed such factors as age, number of previous offenses, and type of crime. Despite the formula's crudeness, it predicted the occurrence of parole violations far more accurately than the psychiatrists did. In recent articles, Meehl and the social scientists David Faust and Robyn Dawes have reviewed more than a hundred studies comparing computers or statistical formulas with human judgment in predicting everything from the likelihood that a company will go bankrupt to the life expectancy of liver-disease patients. In virtually all cases, statistical thinking equaled or surpassed human judgment. You might think that a human being and a computer working together would make the best decisions. But, as the researchers point out, this claim makes little sense. If opinions agree, no matter. If they disagree, the studies show that you're better off sticking with the computer's judgment.

What accounts for the superiority of a well-developed computer algorithm? First, Dawes notes, human beings are inconsistent: we are easily influenced by suggestion, the order in which we see things, recent experience, distractions, and the way information is framed. Second, human beings are not good at considering multiple factors. We tend to give some variables too much weight and wrongly ignore others. A good computer program consistently and automatically gives each factor its appropriate weight. After all, Meehl asks, when we go to the store, do we let the clerk eyeball our groceries and say, "Well, it looks like seventeen dollars' worth to me"? With lots of training, the clerk might get very good at guessing. But we recognize the fact that a computer that simply adds up the prices will be more consistent and more accurate. In the Swedish study, as it turned out, Ohlin rarely made obvious mistakes. But many EKGs are in the gray zone, with some features suggesting a healthy heart and others suggesting a heart attack. Doctors have difficulty estimating faithfully which way the mass of information tips, and they are easily influenced by extraneous factors, such as what the last EKG they came across looked like.

It is probably inevitable that physicians will have to let computers take over at least some diagnostic decisions. One network, PAPNET, has already gained mainstream use in the screening of digitized Pap smears—microscopic scrapings taken from a woman's cervix— for cancer or precancerous abnormalities, which is a job usually done by a pathologist. Researchers have completed more than a thousand studies on the use of neural networks in nearly every field of medicine. Networks have been developed to diagnose appendicitis, dementia, psychiatric emergencies, and sexually transmitted diseases. Others can predict success from cancer treatment, organ transplantation, and heart valve surgery. Systems have been designed to read chest X rays, mammograms, and nuclear-medicine heart scans.

In the treatment of disease, parts of the medical world have already begun to extend the lesson of the Shouldice Hospital concerning the advantages of specialized, automated care. Regina Herzlinger, a professor at the Harvard Business School, who introduced the term "health-care focused factory" in her book *Market-Driven Health Care*, points to other examples, including the Texas Heart Institute for cardiac surgery and Duke University's bone-marrow transplant center. Breast cancer patients seem to do best in specialized cancer treatment centers, where they have a cancer surgeon, an oncologist, a radiation therapist, a plastic surgeon, a social worker, a nutritionist, and others who see breast cancer day in and day out. And almost any hospital one goes to now has protocols and algorithms for treating at least a few common conditions, such as asthma or sudden stroke. The new artificial neural networks merely extend these lessons to the realm of diagnosis.

Still, resistance to this vision of mechanized medicine will remain. Part of it may well be short-sightedness: doctors can be stubborn about changing the way we do things. Part of it, however, stems from legitimate concern that, for all the technical virtuosity gained, something vital is lost in medicine by machine. Modern care already lacks the human touch, and its technocratic ethos has alienated many of the people it seeks to serve. Patients feel like a number too often as it is.

Yet compassion and technology aren't necessarily incompatible; they can be mutually reinforcing. Which is to say that the machine, oddly enough, may be medicine's best friend. On the simplest level, nothing comes between patient and doctor like a mistake. And while errors will always dog us—even machines are not perfect—trust can only increase when mistakes are reduced. Moreover, as "systems" take on more and more of the technical work of medicine, individual physicians may be in a position to embrace the dimensions of care that mattered long before technology came—like talking to their patients. Medical care is about our life and death, and we've always needed doctors to help us understand what is happening and why, and what is possible and what is not. In the increasingly tangled web of experts and expert systems, a doctor has an even greater obligation to serve as a knowledgeable guide and confidant. Maybe machines can decide, but we still need doctors to heal.

When Doctors Make Mistakes

To much of the public—and certainly to lawyers and the media—medical error is fundamentally a problem of bad doctors. The way that things go wrong in medicine is normally unseen and, consequently, often misunderstood. Mistakes do happen. We tend to think of them as aberrant. They are, however, anything but.

At 2 A.M. on a crisp Friday in winter a few years ago, I was in sterile gloves and gown, pulling a teenage knifing victim's abdomen open, when my pager sounded. "Code Trauma, three minutes," the operating room nurse said, reading aloud from my pager display. This meant that an ambulance would be bringing another trauma patient to the hospital momentarily, and, as the surgical resident on duty for emergencies, I would have to be present for the patient's arrival. I stepped back from the table and took off my gown. Two other surgeons were working on the knifing victim: Michael Ball, the attending (the staff surgeon in charge of the case), and David Hernandez, the chief resident (a general surgeon in his final year of training). Ordinarily, these two would have come to supervise and help with the trauma, but they were stuck here. Ball, a dry, cerebral forty-two-year-old, looked over at me as I headed for the door. "If you run into any trouble, you call, and one of us will peel away," he said.

I did run into trouble. In telling this story, I have had to change some details about what happened (including the names of those involved). Nonetheless, I have tried to stay as close to the actual events as I could while protecting the patient, myself, and the rest of the staff.

The emergency room was one floor up, and, taking the stairs two at a time, I arrived just as the emergency medical technicians wheeled in a woman who appeared to be in her thirties and to weigh more than two hundred pounds. She lay motionless on a hard orange plastic spinal board—eyes closed, skin pale, blood running out of her nose. A nurse directed the crew into Trauma Bay 1, an examination room outfitted like an OR, with green tiles on the wall, monitoring devices, and space for portable X-ray equipment. We lifted her onto the bed and then went to work. One nurse began cutting off the woman's clothes. Another took vital signs. A third inserted a large-bore intravenous line into her right arm. A surgical intern put a Foley catheter into her bladder. The emergency-medicine attending was Samuel Johns, a gaunt, Ichabod Crane–like man in his fifties. He was standing to one side with his arms crossed, observing, which was a sign that I could go ahead and take charge.

In an academic hospital, residents provide most of the "moment to moment" doctoring. Our duties depend on our level of training, but we're never entirely on our own: there's always an attending, who oversees our decisions. That night, since Johns was the attending and was responsible for the patient's immediate management, I took my lead from him. At the same time, he wasn't a surgeon, and so he relied on me for surgical expertise.

"What's the story?" I asked.

An EMT rattled off the details: "Unidentified white female unrestrained driver in high-speed rollover. Ejected from the car.

Found unresponsive to pain. Pulse a hundred, BP a hundred over sixty, breathing at thirty on her own . . ."

As he spoke, I began examining her. The first step in caring for a trauma patient is always the same. It doesn't matter if a person has been shot eleven times or crushed by a truck or burned in a kitchen fire. The first thing you do is make sure that the patient can breathe without difficulty. This woman's breaths were shallow and rapid. An oximeter, by means of a sensor placed on her finger, measured the oxygen saturation of her blood. The "O2 sat" is normally more than 95 percent for a patient breathing room air. The woman was wearing a face mask with oxygen turned up full blast, and her sat was only 90 percent.

"She's not oxygenating well," I announced in the flattened-out, wake-me-up-when-something-interesting-happens tone that all surgeons have acquired by about three months into residency. With my fingers, I verified that there wasn't any object in her mouth that would obstruct her airway; with a stethoscope, I confirmed that neither lung had collapsed. I got hold of a bag mask, pressed its clear facepiece over her nose and mouth, and squeezed the bellows, a kind of balloon with a one-way valve, shooting a liter of air into her with each compression. After a minute or so, her oxygen came up to a comfortable 98 percent. She obviously needed our help with breathing. "Let's tube her," I said. That meant putting a tube down through her vocal cords and into her trachea, which would insure a clear airway and allow for mechanical ventilation.

Johns, the attending, wanted to do the intubation. He picked up a Mac 3 laryngoscope, a standard but fairly primitive-looking L-shaped metal instrument for prying open the mouth and throat, and slipped the shoehornlike blade deep into her mouth and down to her larynx. Then he yanked the handle up toward the ceiling to pull her tongue out of the way, open her mouth and throat, and reveal the vocal cords, which sit like fleshy tent flaps at the entrance to the trachea. The patient didn't wince or gag: she was still out cold.

"Suction!" he called. "I can't see a thing."

He sucked out about a cup of blood and clot. Then he picked up the endotracheal tube—a clear rubber pipe about the diameter of an index finger and three times as long—and tried to guide it between her cords. After a minute, her sat started to fall.

"You're down to seventy percent," a nurse announced.

Johns kept struggling with the tube, trying to push it in, but it banged vainly against the cords. The patient's lips began to turn blue.

"Sixty percent," the nurse said.

Johns pulled everything out of the patient's mouth and fitted the bag mask back on. The oximeter's luminescent-green readout hovered at 60 for a moment and then rose steadily, to 97 percent. After a few minutes, he took the mask off and again tried to get the tube in. There was more blood, and there may have been some swelling, too: all the poking down the throat was probably not helping. The sat fell to 60 percent. He pulled out and "bagged" her until she returned to 95 percent.

When you're having trouble getting the tube in, the next step is to get specialized expertise. "Let's call anesthesia," I said, and Johns agreed. In the meantime, I continued to follow the standard trauma protocol: completing the examination and ordering fluids, lab tests, and X rays. Maybe five minutes passed as I worked.

The patient's sats drifted down to 92 percent—not a dramatic change but definitely not normal for a patient who is being manually ventilated. I checked to see if the sensor had slipped off her finger. It hadn't. "Is the oxygen up full blast?" I asked a nurse.

"It's up all the way," she said.

I listened again to the patient's lungs—no collapse. "We've got to get her tubed," Johns said. He took off the oxygen mask and tried again.

Somewhere in my mind, I must have been aware of the possibility that her airway was shutting down because of vocal cord swelling or blood. If it was, and we were unable to get a tube in, then the only chance she'd have to survive would be an emergency tracheotomy: cutting a hole in her neck and inserting a breathing tube into her trachea. Another attempt to intubate her might even trigger a spasm of the cords and a sudden closure of the airway—which is exactly what did happen.

If I had actually thought this far along, I would have recognized how ill-prepared I was to do an emergency "trache." As the one surgeon in the room, it's true, I had the most experience doing tracheotomies, but that wasn't saying much. I had been the assistant surgeon in only about half a dozen, and all but one of them had been non-emergency cases, employing techniques that were not designed for speed. The exception was a practice emergency trache I had done on a goat. I should have immediately called Dr. Ball for backup. I should have got the trache equipment out—lighting, suction, sterile instruments—just in case. Instead of hurrying the effort to get the patient intubated because of a mild drop in saturation, I should have asked Johns to wait until I had help nearby. I might even have recognized that she was already losing her airway. Then I could have grabbed a knife and done a tracheotomy while things were still relatively stable and I had time to proceed slowly. But for whatever reasons—hubris, inattention, wishful thinking, hesitation, or the uncertainty of the moment—I let the opportunity pass.

Johns hunched over the patient, trying intently to insert the tube through her vocal cords. When her sat once again dropped into the 60s, he stopped and put the mask back on. We stared at the monitor. The numbers weren't coming up. Her lips were still blue. Johns squeezed the bellows harder to blow more oxygen in.

"I'm getting resistance," he said.

The realization crept over me: this was a disaster. "Damn it, we've lost her airway," I said. "Trache kit! Light! Somebody call down to OR 25 and get Ball up here!"

People were suddenly scurrying everywhere. I tried to proceed deliberately, and not let panic take hold. I told the surgical intern to get a sterile gown and gloves on. I took an antiseptic solution off a shelf and dumped a whole bottle of yellow-brown liquid on the patient's neck. A nurse unwrapped the tracheostomy kit—a sterilized set of drapes and instruments. I pulled on a gown and a new pair of gloves while trying to think through the steps. This is simple, really, I tried to tell myself. At the base of the thyroid cartilage, the Adam's apple, is a little gap in which you find a thin, fibrous covering called the cricothyroid membrane. Cut through that and—*voilà!* You're in the trachea. You slip through the hole a four-inch plastic tube shaped like a plumber's elbow joint, hook it up to oxygen and a ventilator, and she's all set. Anyway, that was the theory.

I threw some drapes over her body, leaving the neck exposed. It looked as thick as a tree. I felt for the bony prominence of the thyroid cartilage. But I couldn't feel anything through the layers of fat. I was beset by uncertainty—where should I cut? should I make a horizontal or a vertical incision?—and I hated myself for it. Surgeons never dithered, and I was dithering.

"I need better light," I said.

Someone was sent out to look for one.

"Did anyone get Ball?" I asked. It wasn't exactly an inspiring question.

"He's on his way," a nurse said.

There was no time to wait. Four minutes without oxygen would lead to permanent brain damage, if not death. Finally, I took the scalpel and cut. I just cut. I made a three-inch left-to-right swipe across the middle of the neck, following the procedure I'd learned for elective cases. Dissecting down with scissors while the intern held the wound open with retractors, I hit a vein. It didn't let loose a lot of blood, but there was enough to fill the wound: I couldn't see anything. The intern put a finger on the bleeder. I called for suction. But the suction wasn't working; the tube was clogged with clot from the intubation efforts.

"Somebody get some new tubing," I said. "And where's the light?"

Finally, an orderly wheeled in a tall overhead light, plugged it in, and flipped on the switch. It was still too dim; I could have done better with a flashlight.

I wiped up the blood with gauze, then felt around in the wound with my fingertips. This time, I thought I could feel the hard ridges of the thyroid cartilage and, below it, the slight gap of the cricothyroid membrane, though I couldn't be sure. I held my place with my left hand.

James O'Connor, a silver-haired, seen-it-all anesthesiologist, came into the room. Johns gave him a quick rundown on the patient and let him take over ventilating her.

Holding the scalpel in my right hand like a pen, I stuck the blade down into the wound at the spot where I thought the thyroid cartilage was. With small, sharp strokes—working blindly, because of the blood and the poor light—I cut down through the overlying fat and tissue until I felt the blade scrape against the almost bony cartilage. I searched with the tip of the knife, walking it along until I felt it reach a gap. I hoped it was the cricothyroid membrane, and pressed down firmly. I felt the tissue suddenly give, and I cut an inch-long opening.

When I put my index finger into it, it felt as if I were prying open the jaws of a stiff clothespin. Inside, I thought I felt open space. But where were the sounds of moving air that I expected? Was this deep enough? Was I even in the right place?

"I think I'm in," I said, to reassure myself as much as anyone else.

"I hope so," O'Connor said. "She doesn't have much longer."

I took the tracheostomy tube and tried to fit it in, but something seemed to be blocking it. I twisted it and turned it, and finally jammed it in. Just then Ball, the surgical attending, arrived. He rushed up to the bed and leaned over for a look. "Did you get it?" he asked. I said that I thought so. The bag mask was plugged onto the open end of the trache tube. But when the bellows were compressed the air just gurgled out of the wound. Ball quickly put on gloves and a gown.

"How long has she been without an airway?" he asked.

"I don't know. Three minutes."

Ball's face hardened as he registered that he had about a minute in which to turn things around. He took my place and summarily pulled out the trache tube. "God, what a mess," he said. "I can't see a thing in this wound. I don't even know if you're in the right place. Can we get better light and suction?" New suction tubing was found and handed to him. He quickly cleaned up the wound and went to work.

The patient's sat had dropped so low that the oximeter couldn't detect it anymore. Her heart rate began slowing down—first to the 60s and then to the 40s. Then she lost her pulse entirely. I put my hands together on her chest, locked my elbows, leaned over her, and started doing chest compressions.

Ball looked up from the patient and turned to O'Connor. "I'm not going to get her an airway in time," he said. "You're going to have to try again from above." Essentially, he was admitting my failure. Trying an oral intubation again was pointless—just something to do instead of watching her die. I was stricken, and concentrated on doing chest compressions, not looking at anyone. It was over, I thought.

And then, amazingly, O'Connor: "I'm in." He had managed to slip a pediatric-size endotracheal tube through the vocal cords. In thirty seconds, with oxygen being manually ventilated through the tube, her heart was back, racing at a hundred and twenty beats a minute. Her sat registered at 60 and then climbed. Another thirty seconds and it was at 97 percent. All the people in the room exhaled, as if they, too, had been denied their breath. Ball and I said little except to confer about the next steps for her. Then he went back downstairs to finish working on the stab-wound patient still in the OR.

We eventually identified the woman, whom I'll call Louise Williams; she was thirty-four years old and lived alone in a nearby suburb. Her alcohol level on arrival had been three times the legal limit, and had probably contributed to her unconsciousness. She had a concussion, several lacerations, and significant soft-tissue damage. But X rays and scans revealed no other injuries from the crash. That night, Ball and Hernandez brought her to the OR to fit her with a proper tracheostomy. When Ball came out and talked to family members, he told them of the dire condition she was in when she arrived, the difficulties "we" had had getting access to her airway, the disturbingly long period of time that she had gone without oxygen, and thus his uncertainty about how much brain function she still possessed. They listened without protest; there was nothing for them to do but wait.

Consider some other surgical mishaps. In one, a general surgeon left a large metal instrument in a patient's abdomen, where it tore through the bowel and the wall of the bladder. In another, a cancer surgeon biopsied the wrong part of a woman's breast and thereby delayed her diagnosis of cancer for months. A cardiac surgeon skipped a small but key step during a heart valve operation, thereby killing the patient. A general surgeon saw a man racked with abdominal pain in the emergency room and, without taking a CT scan, assumed that the man had a kidney stone; eighteen hours later, a scan showed a rupturing abdominal aortic aneurysm, and the patient died not long afterward.

How could anyone who makes a mistake of that magnitude be allowed to practice medicine? We call such doctors "incompetent," "unethical," and "negligent." We want to see them punished. And so we've wound up with the public system we have for dealing with error: malpractice lawsuits, media scandal, suspensions, firings.

There is, however, a central truth in medicine that complicates this tidy vision of misdeeds and misdoers: all doctors make terrible mistakes. Consider the cases I've just described. I gathered them simply by asking respected surgeons I know—surgeons at top medical schools—to tell me about mistakes they had made just in the past year. Every one of them had a story to tell.

In 1991, the *New England Journal of Medicine* published a series of landmark papers from a project known as the Harvard Medical Practice Study—a review of more than thirty thousand hospital admissions in New York State. The study found that nearly 4 percent of hospital patients suffered complications from treatment which either prolonged their hospital stay or resulted in disability or death, and that two-thirds of such complications were due to errors in care. One in four, or 1 percent of admissions, involved actual negligence. It was estimated that, nationwide, upward of forty-four thousand patients die each year at least partly as a result of errors in care. And subsequent investigations around the country have confirmed the ubiquity of error. In one small study of how clinicians perform when patients have a sudden cardiac arrest, twenty-seven of thirty clinicians made an error in using the defibrillator—charging it incorrectly or losing too much time trying to figure out how to work a particular model. According to a 1995 study, mistakes in administering drugs—giving the wrong drug or the wrong dose, say—occur, on average, about once every hospital admission, mostly without ill effects, but 1 percent of the time with serious consequences.

If error were due to a subset of dangerous doctors, you might expect malpractice cases to be concentrated among a small group, but in fact they follow a uniform, bell-shaped distribution. Most surgeons are sued at least once in the course of their careers. Studies of specific types of error, too, have found that repeat offenders are not the problem. The fact is that virtually everyone who cares for hospital patients will make serious mistakes, and even commit acts of negligence, every year. For this reason, doctors are seldom outraged when the press reports yet another medical horror story. They usually have a different reaction: That could be me. The important question isn't how to keep bad physicians from harming patients; it's how to keep good physicians from harming patients.

Medical malpractice suits are a remarkably ineffective remedy. Troyen Brennan, a Harvard professor of law and public health, points out that research has consistently failed to find evidence that litigation reduces medical error rates. In part, this may be because the weapon is so imprecise. Brennan led several studies following up on the patients in the Harvard Medical Practice Study. He found that fewer than 2 percent of the patients who had received substandard care ever filed suit. Conversely, only a small minority among the patients who did sue had in fact been the victims of negligent care. And a patient's likelihood of winning a suit depended primarily on how poor his or her outcome was, regardless of whether that outcome was caused by disease or unavoidable risks of care.

The deeper problem with medical malpractice suits is that by demonizing errors they prevent doctors from acknowledging and discussing them publicly. The tort system makes adversaries of patient and physician, and pushes each to offer a heavily slanted version of events. When things go wrong, it's almost impossible for a physician to talk to a patient honestly about mistakes. Hospital lawyers warn doctors that, although they must, of course, tell patients about injuries that occur, they are never to intimate that they were at fault, lest the "confession" wind up in court as damning evidence in a black-and-white morality tale. At most, a doctor might say, "I'm sorry that things didn't go as well as we had hoped."

There is one place, however, where doctors can talk candidly about their mistakes, if not with patients, then at least with one another. It is called the Morbidity and Mortality Conference—or, more simply, M & M—and it takes place, usually once a week, at nearly every academic hospital in the country. This institution survives because laws protecting its proceedings from legal discovery have stayed on the books in most states, despite frequent challenges. Surgeons, in particular, take the M & M seriously. Here they can gather behind closed doors to review the mistakes, untoward events, and deaths that occurred on their watch, determine responsibility, and figure out what to do differently next time.

At my hospital, we convene every Tuesday at five o'clock in a steep, plush amphitheater lined with oil portraits of the great doctors whose achievements we're meant to live up to. All surgeons are expected to attend, from the interns to the chairman of surgery; we're also joined by medical students doing their surgery "rotation." An M & M can include almost a hundred people. We file in, pick up a photocopied list of cases to be discussed, and take our seats. The front row is occupied by the most senior surgeons: terse, serious men, now out of their scrubs and in dark suits, lined up like a panel of senators at a hearing. The chairman is a leonine presence in the seat closest to the plain wooden podium from which each case is presented. In the next few rows are the remaining surgical attendings; these tend to be younger, and several of them are women. The chief residents have put on long white coats and usually sit in the side rows. I join the mass of other residents, all of us in short white coats and green scrub pants, occupying the back rows.

For each case, the chief resident from the relevant service — cardiac, vascular, trauma, and so on — gathers the information, takes the podium, and tells the story. Here's a partial list of cases from a typical week (with a few changes to protect confidentiality): a sixty-eight-year-old man who bled to death after heart valve surgery; a forty-seven-year-old woman who had to have a reoperation because of infection following an arterial bypass done in her left leg; a forty-four-year-old woman who had to have bile drained from her abdomen after gallbladder surgery; three patients who had to have reoperations for bleeding following surgery; a sixty-three-year-old man who had a cardiac arrest following heart bypass surgery; a sixty-six-year-old woman whose sutures suddenly gave way in an abdominal wound and nearly allowed her intestines to spill out. Ms. Williams's case, my failed tracheostomy, was just one case on a list like this. David Hernandez, the chief trauma resident, had subsequently reviewed the records and spoken to me and others involved. When the time came, it was he who stood up front and described what had happened.

Hernandez is a tall, rollicking, good old boy who can spin a yarn, but M & M presentations are bloodless and compact. He said something like: "This was a thirty-four-year-old female unrestrained driver in a high-speed rollover. The patient apparently had stable vitals at the scene but was unresponsive, and was brought in by ambulance unintubated. She was GCS 7 on arrival." GCS stands for the Glasgow Coma Scale, which rates the severity of head injuries, from three to fifteen. GCS 7 is in the comatose range. "Attempts to intubate were made without success in the ER and may have contributed to airway closure. A cricothyroidotomy was attempted without success."

These presentations can be awkward. The chief residents, not the attendings, determine which cases to report. That keeps the attendings honest—no one can cover up mistakes—but it puts the chief residents, who are, after all, underlings, in a delicate position. The successful M & M presentation inevitably involves a certain elision of detail and a lot of passive verbs. No one screws up a cricothyroidotomy. Instead, "a cricothyroidotomy was attempted without success." The message, however, was not lost on anyone.

Hernandez continued, "The patient arrested and required cardiac compressions. Anesthesia was then able to place a pediatric ET tube and the patient recovered stable vitals. The tracheostomy was then completed in the OR."

So Louise Williams had been deprived of oxygen long enough to go into cardiac arrest, and everyone knew that meant she could easily have suffered a disabling stroke or worse. Hernandez concluded with the fortunate aftermath: "Her workup was negative for permanent cerebral damage or other major injuries. The tracheostomy tube was removed on Day 2. She was discharged to home in good condition on Day 3." To the family's great relief, and mine, she had woken up in the morning a bit woozy but hungry, alert, and mentally intact. In a few weeks, the episode would heal to a scar.

But not before someone was called to account. A front-row voice immediately thundered, "What do you mean, 'a cricothyroidotomy was attempted without success'?" I sank into my seat, my face hot.

"This was my case," Dr. Ball volunteered from the front row. It is how every attending begins, and that little phrase contains a world of surgical culture. For all the talk in business schools and in corporate America about the virtues of "flat organizations," surgeons maintain an old-fashioned sense of hierarchy. When things go wrong, the attending is expected to take full responsibility. It makes no difference whether it was the resident's hand that slipped and lacerated an aorta; it doesn't matter whether the attending was at home in bed when a nurse gave a wrong dose of medication. At the M & M, the burden of responsibility falls on the attending.

Ball went on to describe the emergency attending's failure to intubate Williams and his own failure to be at her bedside when things got out of control. He described the bad lighting and her extremely thick neck, and was careful to make those sound not like excuses but merely like complicating factors. Some attendings shook their heads in sympathy. A couple of them asked questions to clarify certain details. Throughout, Ball's tone was objective, detached. He had the air of a CNN newscaster describing unrest in Kuala Lumpur.

As always, the chairman, responsible for the overall quality of our surgery service, asked the final question. What, he wanted to know, would Ball have done differently? Well, Ball replied, it didn't take long to get the stab-wound patient under control in the OR, so he probably should have sent Hernandez up to the ER at that point or let Hernandez close the abdomen while he himself came up. People nodded. Lesson learned. Next case.

At no point during the M & M did anyone question why I had not called for help sooner or why I had not had the skill and knowledge that Williams needed. This is not to say that my actions were seen as acceptable. Rather, in the hierarchy, addressing my errors was Ball's role. The day after the disaster, Ball had caught me in the hall and taken me aside. His voice was more wounded than angry as he went through my specific failures. First, he explained, in an emergency tracheostomy it might have been better to do a vertical neck incision; that would have kept me out of the blood vessels, which run up and down—something I should have known at least from my reading. I might have had a much easier time getting her an airway then, he said. Second, and worse to him than mere ignorance, he didn't understand why I hadn't called him when there were clear signs of airway trouble developing. I offered no excuses. I promised to be better prepared for such cases and to be quicker to ask for help.

Even after Ball had gone down the fluorescent-lit hallway, I felt a sense of shame like a burning ulcer. This was not guilt: guilt is what you feel when you have done something wrong. What I felt was shame: I was what was wrong. And yet I also knew that a surgeon can take such feelings too far. It is one thing to be aware of one's limitations. It is another to be plagued by self-doubt. One surgeon with a national reputation told me about an abdominal operation in which he had lost control of bleeding while he was removing what turned out to be a benign tumor and the patient had died. "It was a clean kill," he said. Afterward, he could barely bring himself to operate. When he did operate, he became tentative and indecisive. The case affected his performance for months.

Even worse than losing self-confidence, though, is reacting defensively. There are surgeons who will see faults everywhere except in themselves. They have no questions and no fears about their abilities. As a result, they learn nothing from their mistakes and know nothing of their limitations. As one surgeon told me, it is a rare but alarming thing to meet a surgeon without fear. "If you're not a little afraid when you operate," he said, "you're bound to do a patient a grave disservice."

The atmosphere at the M & M is meant to discourage both attitudes—self-doubt and denial—for the M & M is a cultural ritual that inculcates in surgeons a "correct" view of mistakes. "What would you do differently?" a chairman asks concerning cases of avoidable harm. "Nothing" is seldom an acceptable answer.

In its way, the M & M is an impressively sophisticated and human institution. Unlike the courts or the media, it recognizes that human error is generally not something that can be deterred by punishment. The M & M sees avoiding error as largely a matter of will—of staying sufficiently informed and alert to anticipate the myriad ways that things can go wrong and then trying to head off each potential problem before it happens. It isn't damnable that an error occurs, but there is some shame to it. In fact, the M & M's ethos can seem paradoxical. On the one hand, it reinforces the very American idea that error is intolerable. On the other hand, the very existence of the M & M, its place on the weekly schedule, amounts to an acknowledgment that mistakes are an inevitable part of medicine.

But why do they happen so often? Lucian Leape, medicine's leading expert on error, points out that many other industries— whether the task is manufacturing semiconductors or serving customers at the Ritz-Carlton—simply wouldn't countenance error rates like those in hospitals. The aviation industry has reduced the frequency of operational errors to one in a hundred thousand flights, and most of those errors have no harmful consequences. The buzzword at General Electric these days is "Six Sigma," meaning that its goal is to make product defects so rare that in statistical terms they are more than six standard deviations away from being a matter of chance—almost a one-in-a-million occurrence.

Of course, patients are far more complicated and idiosyncratic than airplanes, and medicine isn't a matter of delivering a fixed product or even a catalogue of products; it may well be more complex than just about any other field of human endeavor. Yet everything we've learned in the past two decades—from cognitive psychology, from "human factors" engineering, from studies of disasters like Three Mile Island and Bhopal—has yielded the same insights: not only do all human beings err, but they err frequently and in predictable, patterned ways. And systems that do not adjust for these realities can end up exacerbating rather than eliminating error.

The British psychologist James Reason argues, in his book *Human Error*, that our propensity for certain types of error is the price we pay for the brain's remarkable ability to think and act intuitively—to sift quickly through the sensory information that constantly bombards us without wasting time trying to work through every situation anew. Thus systems that rely on human perfection present what Reason calls "latent errors"—errors waiting to happen. Medicine teems with examples. Take writing out a prescription, a rote procedure that relies on memory and attention, which we know are unreliable. Inevitably, a physician will sometimes specify the wrong dose or the wrong drug. Even when the prescription is written correctly, there's a risk that it will be misread. (Computerized ordering systems can almost eliminate errors of this kind, but only a small minority of hospitals have adopted them.) Medical equipment, which manufacturers often build without human operators in mind, is another area rife with latent errors: one reason physicians are bound to have problems when they use cardiac defibrillators is that the devices have no standard design. You can also make the case that onerous workloads, chaotic environments, and inadequate team communication all represent latent errors in the system.

James Reason makes another important observation: disasters do not simply occur; they evolve. In complex systems, a single failure rarely leads to harm. Human beings are impressively good at adjusting when an error becomes apparent, and systems often have built-in defenses. For example, pharmacists and nurses routinely check and countercheck physicians' orders. But errors do not always become apparent, and backup systems themselves often fail as a result of latent errors. A pharmacist forgets to check one of a thousand prescriptions. A machine's alarm bell malfunctions. The one attending trauma surgeon available gets stuck in the operating room. When things go wrong, it is usually because a series of failures conspires to produce disaster.

The M & M takes none of this into account. For that reason, many experts see it as a rather shabby approach to analyzing error and improving performance in medicine. It isn't enough to ask what a clinician could or should have done differently so that he and others may learn for next time. The doctor is often only the final actor in a chain of events that set him or her up to fail. Error experts, therefore, believe that it's the process, not the individuals in it, that requires closer examination and correction. In a sense, they want to industrialize medicine. And they can already claim successes: the Shouldice Hospital's "focused factory" for hernia operations, for one—and far more broadly, the entire specialty of anesthesiology, which has adopted their precepts and seen extraordinary results.

At the center of the emblem of the American Society of Anesthesiologists is a single word: "Vigilance." When you put a patient to sleep under general anesthesia, you assume almost complete control of the patient's body. The body is paralyzed, the brain rendered unconscious, and machines are hooked up to control breathing, heart rate, blood pressure—all the vital functions. Given the complexity of the machinery and of the human body, there are a seemingly infinite number of ways in which things can go wrong, even in minor surgery. And yet anesthesiologists have found that if problems are detected they can usually be solved. In the 1940s, there was only one death resulting from anesthesia in every twenty-five hundred operations, and between the 1960s and the 1980s the rate had stabilized at one or two in every ten thousand operations.

But Ellison (Jeep) Pierce had always regarded even that rate as unconscionable. From the time he began practicing, in 1960, as a young anesthesiologist out of North Carolina and the University of

Pennsylvania, he had maintained a case file of details from all the deadly anesthetic accidents he had come across or participated in. But it was one case in particular that galvanized him. Friends of his had taken their eighteen-year-old daughter to the hospital to have her wisdom teeth pulled, under general anesthesia. The anesthesiologist inserted the breathing tube into her esophagus instead of her trachea, which is a relatively common mishap, and then failed to spot the error, which is not. Deprived of oxygen, she died within minutes. Pierce knew that a one-in-ten-thousand death rate, given that anesthesia was administered in the United States an estimated thirty-five million times each year, meant thirty-five hundred avoidable deaths like that one.

In 1982, Pierce was elected vice president of the American Society of Anesthesiologists and got an opportunity to do something about the death rate. The same year, ABC's 20/20 aired an exposé that caused a considerable stir in his profession. The segment began, "If you are going to go into anesthesia, you are going on a long trip, and you should not do it if you can avoid it in any way. General anesthesia [is] safe most of the time, but there are dangers from human error, carelessness, and a critical shortage of anesthesiologists. This year, six thousand patients will die or suffer brain damage." The program presented several terrifying cases from around the country. Between the small crisis that the show created and the sharp increases in physicians' malpractice insurance premiums at that time, Pierce was able to mobilize the Society of Anesthesiologists to focus on the problem of error.

He turned for ideas not to a physician but to an engineer named Jeffrey Cooper, the lead author of a groundbreaking 1978 paper entitled "Preventable Anesthesia Mishaps: A Study of Human Factors." An unassuming, fastidious man, Cooper had been hired in 1972, when he was twenty-six years old, by the Massachusetts General Hospital bioengineering unit, to work on developing machines for anesthesiology researchers. He gravitated toward the operating room, however, and spent hours there observing the anesthesiologists, and one of the first things he noticed was how poorly the anesthesia machines were designed. For example, a clockwise turn of a dial decreased the concentration of potent anesthetics in about half the machines but increased the concentration in the other half. He decided to borrow a technique called "critical incident analysis"— which had been used since the 1950s to analyze mishaps in aviation—in an effort to learn how equipment might be contributing to errors in anesthesia. The technique is built around carefully conducted interviews, designed to capture as much detail as possible about dangerous incidents: how specific accidents evolved and what factors contributed to them. This information is then used to look for patterns among different cases.

Getting open, honest reporting is crucial. The Federal Aviation Administration has a formalized system for analyzing and reporting dangerous aviation incidents, and its enormous success in improving airline safety rests on two cornerstones. Pilots who report an incident within ten days have automatic immunity from punishment, and the reports go to a neutral, outside agency, NASA, which has no interest in using the information against individual pilots. For Jeffrey Cooper, it was probably an advantage that he was an engineer and not a physician, so that anesthesiologists regarded him as a discreet, unthreatening researcher.

The result was the first in-depth scientific look at errors in medicine. His detailed analysis of three hundred and fifty-nine errors provided a view of the profession unlike anything that had been seen before. Contrary to the prevailing assumption that the start of anesthesia ("takeoff") was the most dangerous part, anesthesiologists learned that incidents tended to occur in the middle of anesthesia, when vigilance waned. The most common kind of incident involved errors in maintaining the patient's breathing, and these were usually the result of an undetected disconnection or misconnection of the breathing tubing, mistakes in managing the airway, or mistakes in using the anesthesia machine. Just as important, Cooper enumerated a list of contributory factors, including inadequate experience, inadequate familiarity with equipment, poor communication among team members, haste, inattention, and fatigue.

The study provoked widespread debate among anesthesiologists, but there was no concerted effort to solve the problems until Jeep Pierce came along. Through the anesthesiology society at first, and then through a foundation that he started, Pierce directed funding into research on how to reduce the problems Cooper had identified, sponsored an international conference to gather ideas from around the world, and brought anesthesia machine designers into safety discussions.

It all worked. Hours for anesthesiology residents were shortened. Manufacturers began redesigning their machines with fallible human beings in mind. Dials were standardized to turn in a uniform direction; locks were put in to prevent accidental administration of more than one anesthetic gas; controls were changed so that oxygen delivery could not be turned down to zero.

Where errors could not be eliminated directly, anesthesiologists began looking for reliable means of detecting them earlier. For example, because the trachea and the esophagus are so close together, it is almost inevitable that an anesthesiologist will sometimes put the breathing tube down the wrong pipe. Anesthesiologists had always checked for this by listening with a stethoscope for breath sounds over both lungs. But Cooper had turned up a surprising number of mishaps—like the one that befell the daughter of Pierce's friends—involving undetected esophageal intubations. Something more effective was needed. In fact, monitors that could detect this kind of error had been available for years, but, in part because of their expense, relatively few anesthesiologists used them. One type of monitor could verify that the tube was in the trachea by detecting carbon dioxide being exhaled from the lungs. Another type, the pulse oximeter, tracked blood oxygen levels, thereby providing an early warning that something was wrong with the patient's breathing system. Prodded by Pierce and others, the anesthesiology society made the use of both types of monitor for every patient receiving general anesthesia an official standard. Today, anesthesia deaths from misconnecting the breathing system or intubating the esophagus rather than the trachea are virtually unknown. In a decade, the overall death rate dropped to just one in more than two hundred thousand cases—less than a twentieth of what it had been.

And the reformers have not stopped there. David Gaba, a professor of anesthesiology at Stanford, has focused on improving human performance. In aviation, he points out, pilot experience is recognized to be invaluable but insufficient: pilots seldom have direct experience with serious plane malfunctions anymore. They are therefore required to undergo yearly training in crisis simulators. Why not doctors, too?

Gaba, a physician with training in engineering, led in the design of an anesthesia-simulation system known as the Eagle Patient Simulator. It is a life-size, computer-driven mannequin that is capable of amazingly realistic behavior. It has a circulation, a heartbeat, and lungs that take in oxygen and expire carbon dioxide. If you inject drugs into it or administer inhaled anesthetics, it will detect the type and amount, and its heart rate, its blood pressure, and its oxygen levels will respond appropriately. The "patient" can be made to develop airway swelling, bleeding, and heart disturbances. The mannequin is laid on an operating table in a simulation room equipped exactly like the real thing. Here both residents and experienced attending physicians learn to perform effectively in all kinds of dangerous, and sometimes freak, scenarios: an anesthesia machine malfunction, a power outage, a patient who goes into cardiac arrest during surgery, and even a cesarean-section patient whose airway shuts down and who requires an emergency tracheostomy.

Though anesthesiology has unquestionably taken the lead in analyzing and trying to remedy "systems" failures, there are signs of change in other quarters. The American Medical Association, for example, set up its National Patient Safety Foundation in 1997 and asked Cooper and Pierce to serve on the board of directors. The foundation is funding research, sponsoring conferences, and attempting to develop new standards for hospital drug-ordering systems that could substantially reduce medication mistakes—the single most common type of medical error.

Even in surgery there have been some encouraging developments. For instance, operating on the wrong knee or foot or other body part of a patient has been a recurrent, if rare, mistake. A typical response has been to fire the surgeon. Recently, however, hospitals and surgeons have begun to recognize that the body's bilateral symmetry makes these errors predictable. In 1998, the American Academy of Orthopedic Surgeons endorsed a simple way of preventing them: make it standard practice for surgeons to initial, with a marker, the body part to be cut before the patient comes to surgery.

The Northern New England Cardiovascular Disease Study Group, based at Dartmouth, is another success story. Though the group doesn't conduct the sort of in-depth investigation of mishaps that Jeffrey Cooper pioneered, it has shown what can be done simply through statistical monitoring. Six hospitals belong to this consortium, which tracks deaths and other bad outcomes (such as wound infection, uncontrolled bleeding, and stroke) arising from heart surgery and tries to identify the various risk factors involved. Its researchers found, for example, that there were relatively high death rates among patients who developed anemia after bypass surgery, and that anemia developed most often in small patients. The solution used to "prime" the heart-lung machine caused the anemia, because it diluted a patient's blood, so the smaller the patient (and his or her blood supply) the greater the effect. Members of the consortium now have several promising solutions to the problem. Another study found that a group at one hospital had made mistakes in "handoffs"—say, in passing preoperative lab results to the people in the operating room. The study group solved the problem by developing a pilot's checklist for all patients coming to the OR. These efforts have introduced a greater degree of standardization, and so reduced the death rate in those six hospitals from 4 percent to 3 percent between 1991 and 1996. That meant two hundred and ninety-three fewer deaths. But the Northern New England cardiac group, even with its narrow focus and techniques, remains an exception; hard information about how things go wrong is still scarce. There is a hodgepodge of evidence that latent errors and systemic factors may contribute to surgical errors: the lack of standardized protocols, the surgeon's inexperience, the hospital's inexperience, inadequately designed technology and techniques, thin staffing, poor teamwork, time of day, the effects of managed care and corporate medicine, and so on and so on. But which are the major risk factors? We still don't know. Surgery, like most of medicine, awaits its Jeff Cooper.

It was a routine gallbladder operation, on a routine day: on the operating table was a mother in her forties, her body covered by blue paper drapes except for her round, antiseptic-coated belly. The gallbladder is a floppy, finger-length sac of bile like a deflated olive-green balloon tucked under the liver, and when gallstones form, as this patient had learned, they can cause excruciating bouts of pain. Once we removed her gallbladder, the pain would stop.

There are risks to this surgery, but they used to be much greater. Just a decade ago, surgeons had to make a six-inch abdominal incision that left patients in the hospital for the better part of a week just recovering from the wound. Today, we've learned to take out gallbladders with a miniature camera and instruments that we manipulate through tiny incisions. The operation, often done as day surgery, is known as laparoscopic cholecystectomy, or "lap chole." Half a million Americans a year now have their gallbladders removed this way; at my hospital alone, we do several hundred lap choles annually.

When the attending gave me the go-ahead, I cut a discreet inch-long semicircle in the wink of skin just above the belly button. I dissected through fat and fascia until I was inside the abdomen and dropped into place a "port," a half-inch-wide sheath for slipping instruments in and out. We hooked gas tubing up to a side vent on the port, and carbon dioxide poured in, inflating the abdomen until it was distended like a tire. I inserted the miniature camera. On a video monitor a few feet away, the woman's intestines blinked into view. With the abdomen inflated, I had room to move the camera, and I swung it around to look at the liver. The gallbladder could be seen poking out from under the edge.

We put in three more ports through even tinier incisions, spaced apart to complete the four corners of a square. Through the ports on his side, the attending put in two long "graspers," like small-scale versions of the device that a department store clerk might use to get a hat off the top shelf. Watching the screen as he maneuvered them, he reached under the edge of the liver, clamped onto the gallbladder, and pulled it up into view. We were set to proceed.

Removing the gallbladder is fairly straightforward. You sever it from its stalk and from its blood supply, and pull the rubbery sac out of the abdomen through the incision near the belly button. You let the carbon dioxide out of the belly, pull out the ports, put a few stitches in the tiny incisions, slap some Band-Aids on top, and you're done. There's one looming danger, though: the stalk of the gallbladder is a branch off the liver's only conduit for sending bile to the intestines for the digestion of fats. And if you accidentally injure this main bile duct, the bile backs up and starts to destroy the liver. Between 10 and 20 percent of the patients to whom this happens will die. Those who survive often have permanent liver damage and can go on to require liver transplantation. According to a textbook, "Injuries to the main bile duct are nearly always the result of misadventure during operation and are therefore a serious reproach to the surgical profession." It is a true surgical error, and, like any surgical team doing a lap chole, we were intent on avoiding this mistake.

Using a dissecting instrument, I carefully stripped off the fibrous white tissue and yellow fat overlying and concealing the base of the gallbladder. Now we could see its broad neck and the short stretch where it narrowed down to a duct—a tube no thicker than a daisy stem peeking out from the surrounding tissue, but magnified on the screen to the size of major plumbing. Then, just to be absolutely sure we were looking at the gallbladder duct and not the main bile duct, I stripped away some more of the surrounding tissue. The attending and I stopped at this point, as we always do, and discussed the anatomy. The neck of the gallbladder led straight into the tube we were eyeing. So it had to be the right duct. We had exposed a good length of it without a sign of the main bile duct. Everything looked perfect, we agreed. "Go for it," the attending said.

I slipped in the clip applier, an instrument that squeezes V-shaped metal clips onto whatever you put in its jaws. I got the jaws around the duct and was about to fire when my eye caught, on the screen, a little globule of fat lying on top of the duct. That wasn't necessarily anything unusual, but somehow it didn't look right. With the tip of the clip applier, I tried to flick it aside, but instead of a little globule, a whole layer of thin unseen tissue came up, and, underneath, we saw that the duct had a fork in it. My heart dropped. If not for that little extra fastidiousness, I would have clipped off the main bile duct.

Here was the paradox of error in medicine. With meticulous technique and assiduous effort to insure that they have correctly identified the anatomy, surgeons need never cut the main bile duct. It is a paradigm of an avoidable error. At the same time, studies show that even highly experienced surgeons inflict this terrible injury about once in every two hundred lap choles. To put it another way, I may have averted disaster this time, but a statistician would say that, no matter how hard I tried, I was almost certain to make this error at least once in the course of my career.

But the story doesn't have to end here, as the cognitive psychologists and industrial error experts have demonstrated. Given the results they've achieved in anesthesiology, it's clear that we can make dramatic improvements by going after the process, not the people. But there are distinct limitations to the industrial cure, however necessary its emphasis on systems and structures. It would be deadly for us, the individual actors, to give up our belief in human perfectibility. The statistics may say that someday I will sever someone's main bile duct, but each time I go into a gallbladder operation I believe that with enough will and effort I can beat the odds. This isn't just professional vanity. It's a necessary part of good medicine, even in superbly "optimized" systems. Operations like that lap chole have taught me how easily error can occur, but they've also showed me something else: effort does matter; diligence and attention to the minutest details can save you.

This may explain why many doctors take exception to talk of "systems problems," "continuous quality improvement," and "process re-engineering." It is the dry language of structures, not people. I'm no exception: something in me, too, demands an acknowledgment of my autonomy, which is also to say my ultimate culpability. Go back to that Friday night in the ER, to the moment when I stood, knife in hand, over Louise Williams, her lips blue, her throat a swollen, bloody, and suddenly closed passage. A systems engineer might have proposed some useful changes. Perhaps a backup suction device should always be at hand, and better light more easily available. Perhaps the institution could have trained me better for such crises, could have required me to have operated on a few more goats. Perhaps emergency tracheostomies are so difficult under any circumstances that an automated device could have been designed to do a better job.

Yet although the odds were against me, it wasn't as if I had no chance of succeeding. Good doctoring is all about making the most of the hand you're dealt, and I failed to do so. The indisputable fact was that I hadn't called for help when I could have, and when I plunged the knife into her neck and made my horizontal slash my best was not good enough. It was just luck, hers and

Nine Thousand Surgeons

"Are you going to the convention?" the attending asked.

"Me?" I said. He was speaking of the upcoming American College of Surgeons convention. It had never occurred to me that I could go.

Conventions are big deals in medicine. My doctor parents have gone to their conventions faithfully for thirty years, and I vaguely remembered, from the occasions in my childhood when they had brought me along, how dense and enormous and exciting they seemed. As a resident, I had gotten used to the operating schedule suddenly emptying out each mid-October, when the faculty surgeons packed off to their annual convention en masse. But we residents would stay behind, along with a skeleton crew of unlucky attendings (usually the most junior ones), to manage the trauma cases and other random emergencies that still came in. A lot of the time was spent kicked back in the residents' lounge—a dim musty den with flat brown carpeting, a moldering couch, a broken rowing machine, empty soda cans, and two televisions—watching end-of-year baseball on the one television that worked and eating take-out Chinese.

Each year, however, a few senior residents have gotten to tag along to the convention. And in my sixth year I was told that I had now reached the stage in training that allowed me to be one of them. The hospital turned out to have a small fund that would pay for the trip. Within a few days I had a plane ticket to Chicago, a reservation at the Hyatt Regency, and an admission badge for the eighty-sixth annual Clinical Congress of Surgeons. It was not until I was at twenty-seven thousand feet in a Boeing 737 somewhere over New Hampshire, my wife settled back home for a week in sole possession of our three children, that I finally thought to wonder what on earth one goes to these things for.

I arrived at Chicago's massive McCormick Place convention center to find that I was but one of nine thousand three hundred and twelve surgeons in attendance. (A daily newspaper just for the convention reported the daily count.) The building looked like an airport terminal and felt like Penn Station at rush hour. I took an escalator up to a deck above the main hall and looked out upon the sprawl. There were, it struck me, nearly as many people milling around this one building talking surgery as live in the Ohio towns around where I grew up. The surgeons—mostly men and middle-aged, a little shlumpy, in navy jackets, wrinkled shirts, conservative ties—were gathering in clumps of two and three, everyone smiling, shaking hands, catching up. Nearly all wore glasses and stood with a slight operating-table stoop. A few stood alone, leafing through their program books, deciding what to see and do first.

Each of us, upon arriving, had been handed a three hundred and eighty-eight–page schedule of programs we could attend—from a course that first morning on how to do advanced image-guided breast biopsies to a panel presentation on the sixth and final day entitled "Office-Based Treatment of Ano-Rectal Disease—How Far Can We Go?" Eventually, I too settled down with my book, diligently scanning it page by page and circling in blue ballpoint pen anything that caught my eye. This was, I decided, the place where the new and better could be found—the place where the more nearly perfect was being taught—and it seemed almost an obligation to attend as much of the proceedings as I could. Before long my book was blue with circles. The first morning alone, I had more than twenty instructive-looking programs to choose from. I debated going to a lecture on the proper way to dissect a neck or a session on new advances in managing gunshot wounds to the head, but finally decided on a panel debate about the best way to repair hernias of the groin.

I arrived early, and already the auditorium's fifteen hundred seats were filled. Hernias were SRO. I found a place to stand in a crowd along the back wall. I could hardly see the lectern up front, but a giant video screen provided close-ups of each of the talking heads. Eleven surgeons, one after another, took the podium to flash up Powerpoint slides and argue about data.

Our research indicates, the first surgeon intoned, that the Lichtenstein method is the most reliable way to repair hernias. No, the next surgeon rejoined, the Lichtenstein method is inadequate; the Shouldice technique has proven best. Then a third surgeon stepped forward: Both of you are wrong—it should be done laparoscopically. Now another surgeon was up: I've got an even better way to do it, using a special device that I happen to have patented. Things went on this way for two and a half hours. Tempers sometimes flared. Pointed questions were thrown out from the audience. And no answers were reached. But at the end the room was as full as it was at the very beginning.

In the afternoon, I went to the movies. The organizers had set up three theaters seating three or four hundred people each to show reel upon reel of actual operations all day, every day. I scooted into one darkened room and was instantly riveted. I saw daring operations, intricate operations, ingeniously simple operations. The first movie I caught was from Memorial Sloan Kettering Cancer Center in Manhattan. It began with a close-up of a patient's open abdomen. The surgeon, unseen but for his gloved and bloody hands, was attempting an exceedingly difficult and dangerous operation—the excision of a cancer in the tail of a patient's pancreas. The tumor lay deep, enveloped by loops of bowel, a latticework of blood vessels, the stomach, and the spleen. But the surgeon made getting it out seem like play. He plucked at fragile vessels and slashed through tissue millimeters from vital organs. He showed us a couple of tricks for avoiding trouble, and the next thing we knew he had half the pancreas on a tray.

In another film, a team from Strasbourg, France, removed a colon cancer from deep in a patient's pelvis and then reconnected her bowel entirely laparoscopically—through tiny incisions that required only Band-Aids afterward. It was a startling, Houdini-like feat—something akin to removing a model ship from a bottle and constructing a working car in its place using just chopsticks. The audience watched wide-eyed and incredulous.

The most elegant clip, however, was from a Houston, Texas, surgeon who unveiled a procedure for repairing a defect of the esophagus known as Zenker's diverticulum. This is an abnormality that normally requires an hour or more to repair and an incision in the side of the neck, but in the film the surgeon managed to do it through a patient's mouth in fifteen minutes with no incision at all. I stayed and watched movies for almost four hours. And when the lights went up, I walked out into the day silent, blinking, and exhilarated.

The clinical sessions were lined up until 10:30 each night, and they seemed to all go like those first two I attended—veering between the pedantic and the sublime, the mundane and the remarkable. If such programs were supposed to be the meat of the meeting, however, it was often hard to tell. The convention, one soon realized, was as much trade show as teaching conference. Ads for cool new things you had never heard of—a tissue-stapling device that staples without staples, a fiber-optic scope that lets you see in three dimensions—ran night and day on my hotel room television and even on the shuttle bus to and from the convention center. Drug and medical device companies offered invitations to free dinners around town nightly. And there were over five thousand three hundred salespeople from some twelve hundred companies registered in attendance here—more than one for every two surgeons.

The centerpiece of their activity was a teeming, soccer field–size "technical exhibit" hall where they had set up booths from which to market their wares. The word "booth" does not come close to capturing what they had built. There were two-story-high kiosks, pulsing lights, brushed-steel displays, multimedia presentations—one company had even assembled a complete operating room on-site. Surgeons are people who buy two hundred–dollar scissors, sixteen thousand–dollar abdominal retractors, and fifty thousand–dollar operating tables as a matter of course. So the courting can be intense and elaborate.

It was also unavoidable. The convention organizers had given— or more precisely, sold—the salespeople the convention's most prime real estate: their exhibit hall was adjacent to the registration desk, making it the first thing surgeons saw upon arriving at the convention, and our only path to the scientific exhibits was through the glittery maze. Heading through to see a molecular biology exhibit the following afternoon, I never made it to the other side. Everywhere you looked was something to stop you in your tracks.

Sometimes it was just chintzy, free stuff. Booths were offering free golf balls, fountain pens, penlights, baseball caps, sticky pads, candy—all stenciled with company logos, of course, and handed over with a spiel and a brochure about some new technology a company was marketing. You might think six-figure surgeons would be oblivious to this kind of petty bribery. But you would be wrong. A drug manufacturer ran what seemed to be one of the busiest booths in the place handing out sturdy white canvas bags with the name of one of its drugs emblazoned in four-inch blue letters along the side. Doctors lined up for the bags, even when they had to give away their phone numbers and addresses, just to get something to hold all the free merchandise they were collecting. (Still, I heard one physician muttering that the pickings were not as good as in previous years. He'd gotten Ray-Ban sunglasses once, he said.)

Sometimes the companies relied on more subliminal methods to draw surgeons in — putting three smiling young women at a booth, say. "Have you seen our skin?" one leggy brunette with eyelashes like springboards and a voice as vaporous as smoke breathed to me. She meant her company's new artificial skin for burn patients, but how could I resist? The next thing I knew, I was poking with a pair of forceps at an almost translucent white sheet of engineered skin in a petri dish (ninety-five dollars for a four-by-six-inch piece) thinking, "This stuff is pretty neat, actually."

The companies' most effective tactic, however, was simply to put out the goods and let surgeons play. The salespeople would bring out a tray of raw meat and their latest gizmo, and we would flock around like crows. I was sucked in that afternoon by a fresh, yellowy, thirteen-pound turkey on a cookie sheet (cost: about fifteen dollars) and a line of harmonic scalpels (cost: about fifteen thousand dollars) — electronic scalpels that cut through tissue with ultrasonic shock waves. For ten whole and happy minutes, I stood at a glass counter, slicing through layers of turkey skin and muscle, raising thin flaps and thick flaps of tissue, trying deep gouges and intricate dissections, and testing the heft and feel of the various models. At another booth, I donned surgical gloves and tried sewing closed an incision in chicken meat with several lengths of a new fifty-dollar-a-yard suture. I would have stayed throwing knots and practicing my locking stitches for half an hour if four other surgeons hadn't been stacked in line behind me. In the course of the afternoon, I cauterized cold cuts, used advanced laparoscopic equipment to remove "gallstones" — actually, peanut M&Ms — from inside a mannequin's abdomen, and used an automated suturing device to sew closed a wound in a weirdly human-looking piece of flesh. (The salesman was coy and would not tell me what it actually was.)

Having given up totally on making it to anything else that day, I spotted a crowd of some fifty surgeons swarming around a projection screen and a man wearing a suit and a headset microphone. I went up to see what all the fuss was about, and what I found was the live televised image of a patient undergoing excision of a large, prolapsed, internal hemorrhoid in an operating room somewhere, apparently, in Pennsylvania. The manufacturer was showing off a new disposable device (cost: two hundred fifty dollars) that it claimed shortens the usual half-hour procedure to one that takes less than five minutes. The emcee in the headset fielded questions from the crowd which he then put to the surgeon as he operated a thousand miles away.

"You are putting in a purse-string suture now?" the emcee asked.

"Yes," the surgeon replied. "I am putting in the purse-string suture in five or six bites, two centimeters from the base of the hemorrhoids."

Then he put the device before the camera. It was white and shiny and lovely. Against any high-minded desire to stick to hard evidence about whether the technology was actually useful, effective, and reliable, we were all transfixed.

When the show was over, I noticed just a few steps away a forlorn-looking pockfaced man in a rumpled brown suit sitting alone at a tiny booth. People flowed past him like minnows, not one stopping to examine his merchandise. He had no video screens, no brushed-steel displays, no free stenciled golf tees—just a computer-printed logo-less paper sign ("Scientia," it read) and several hundred antiquarian books of surgery. Feeling pity for him, I stopped to browse and was stunned to discover what he had on offer. He had, for example, Joseph Lister's actual 1867 articles in which he had detailed his revolutionary antiseptic method of surgery. He had the first 1924 edition of the great surgeon William Halsted's collected scientific papers and the original 1955 proceedings of the world's first conference on organ transplantation. He had an 1899 catalogue of surgical instruments, a two-centuries-old surgical textbook, and a complete reproduction of a medical text by Maimonides. He even had the 1863 diary of a Union Army Civil War surgeon. There was a trove of jewels in his crates and on his shelves, and I ended up absorbed in them for the rest of the afternoon.

Leafing through those yellowed and brittle pages, I felt I had finally discovered something genuine. Throughout the convention—on the commercial floor, to be sure, but in the lecture halls as well—I noticed myself having to be constantly alert to the possibility that someone was taking me for a ride. There were undoubtedly new drugs and instruments and machines of real and lasting value to be found. With all the glitz and showmanship surrounding them, however, you could never be sure which they were. This was one place where I knew I had found something worthy of awe.

There was another place at the convention where you could be confident of seeing great things going on. Well away from the main halls—where the movies were shown, the practical sessions were held, and the merchandise was hawked—was a cluster of small meeting rooms where the "Surgical Forums" took place. Here each day researchers of all sorts discussed the work they had under way. The subjects ranged from genetics to immunology to physics to population statistics. The discussions were sparsely attended and mostly went over my head: it is impossible nowadays to have a working understanding of even the basic terminology in all of the fields under consideration. But as I sat there listening to the scientists talking among themselves, I caught a glimpse of where the edges of knowledge were, the approachable frontiers.

A recurring topic this year was tissue engineering, a line of research devoted to grasping precisely how organs develop and then using that knowledge to one day grow new organs from scratch that could replace injured or diseased ones. Progress, it became clear, was occurring surprisingly quickly. A couple years before, there had been pictures in all the newspapers of the famous ear grown in a petri dish and implanted on the back of a mouse. But more complex structures, and certainly human trials, seemed a decade or more away. Now, however, scientists were presenting photographs of heart valves, of lengths of blood vessel, and of segments of intestine they had already grown in their laboratories. The problems they discussed were no longer how to do such things but how to do such things better. The heart valves, for example, worked well when experimentally implanted in the hearts of pigs, but didn't last as long as they would need to for humans. Likewise, the intestinal segments proved to be amazingly functional when transplanted into rats, but they did not absorb nutrients as well as desired, and the researchers still had to figure out how to grow them in lengths of feet rather than inches. A team at Cedars-Sinai Hospital in Los Angeles had actually gotten far enough along to begin human trials of a temporary, bioengineered liver.

The researchers presented data from their first dozen patients. Each of the patients had reached the end stage of liver failure, a stage in which 90 percent usually die waiting for a liver transplant. But with the bioengineered liver, the researchers reported, all of them survived long enough to find a donor liver—in many cases ten days or more, which was an unheard-of accomplishment. More remarkably, four patients who had been in end-stage failure from drug overdoses wound up never needing a transplant. The bioengineered liver had kept each going long enough for his or her own liver to recover and regenerate. Sitting in the audience, I experienced a sudden giddiness upon realizing what these doctors had done. And I began to wonder if it was at all like what Joseph Lister's colleagues at the Royal College of Surgeons had felt when he first presented his findings on antisepsis, nearly a century and a half ago.

Was any of this—the teaching, the trade show, the research— what brought thousands of surgeons to spend a week of hard-to-find vacation time in overcast Chicago? There was another convention taking place in town that very same week: the Public Relations

World Congress, "the annual meeting of the planet's public relations professionals." (Theme: "Building Our Talent in a World of Tough Issues.") They too came in droves. Between the surgeons and the flacks, the hotels were booked solid. And our proceedings were almost identical. The publicists had, just as we had, a slew of educational sessions. (Among the events were workshops on managing Internet PR disasters and on starting your own PR firm, as well as a lecture entitled "Conference Calls: A Cost-Effective Tool to Reach Clients and the Press.") They too devoted a full day to research presentations. They had corporate ads everywhere and a lobby filled with exhibits from PR firms, media release services, and the makers of ultrahigh-speed fax machines. Their week closed, just like ours, with a semi-celebrity keynote address. The elements of the conventions were so weirdly alike that you had to think that they were the core of what drew people to come. Wandering the publicists' convention one morning, though, I found their meeting rooms no more than half-filled and the crowds instead out in the halls. Even at our convention, you could sense the enthusiasm for actually learning something quickly wearing thin. By midweek, finding a seat at lectures was no problem. And among those attending, a large chunk either dozed off or left early to stroll the corridors.

The anthropologist Lawrence Cohen describes conferences and conventions not so much as scholarly goings-on but as carnivals— "colossal events where academic proceedings are overshadowed by professional politics, ritual enactments of disciplinary boundaries, sexual liminality, tourism and trade, personal and national rivalries, the care and feeding of professional kinship, and the sheer enormity of discourse." Certainly, in surgery, this seems apt. It did not take long here to realize that some had come just to be seen, others to make their name, still others for the spectacle of it all. There were battles for office (a new president and board of governors were elected) and muckety-mucks meeting behind closed doors. There were residency reunions. There were nights out at Spago and no doubt some love affairs, too.

Yet, true as all of this was, one still had the sense that the draw was deeper than mere carnival. You could see it, for example, on the bus. Every day we surgeons rode back and forth between the convention center and our hotels in fleets of long tour buses. (They were like the ones Greyhound runs to Atlantic City, except ours had drop-down mini-televisions running ads for the "Surgical Zipper.") We were by and large strangers—I never knew anyone on those bus rides—but if you had watched us, it wouldn't have seemed that way. Consider the simple matter of seating. Normally, people boarding a bus, plane, or train distribute themselves like repelling magnets, keeping a respectful, anonymous distance from one another and sharing seats only if they have to. But embarking our buses, we found ourselves choosing to sit two-by-two, even as other seats were empty. Somehow, without anyone saying so, the social rules had been inverted. On any other bus in Chicago, you would have felt almost physically threatened by a stranger sidling up to you when three-quarters of the seats sat empty. Here, however, it would have been the person who set himself apart who provoked the most unease. You were, you felt, among your tribe—connected though knowing no one. You felt the need to say hello. Indeed, it seemed impolite not to do so.

On one shuttle ride, I sat down next to a forty-something-looking man in a blazer and open-collared shirt. We started talking almost immediately. He was, I learned, from a town of thirty-five hundred on the northernmost tip of Michigan's lower peninsula, where he was one of only two general surgeons for fifty miles. Together he and his partner handled everything: pickup-truck crashes, perforated ulcers, appendectomies, colon cancers, breast cancers, even the occasional emergency childbirth. He'd been there for some two decades, he said, and like my parents was a native of India. I was impressed that he had learned to tolerate the winters. I told him of how, almost thirty years before, my parents had narrowed their choices of where to take up practice to either Athens, Ohio, or Hancock, Michigan, in the upper peninsula. Arriving in Hancock by prop plane for a mid-November visit, however, they found three feet of snow already on the ground. Stepping out in her sari, my mother nixed the place immediately and chose Athens, though she had yet to visit it. My seatmate burst out laughing and then said what all deep northerners say about the bitter cold, "Oh, it's really not so bad." Our conversation drifted from weather to our children to my residency to his residency to a piece of laparoscopic equipment he had seen and was thinking of buying. In the seats around us, it was much the same. Bright chatter filled the bus. There were people arguing about baseball (the Mets-Yankees Subway Series was on), politics (Gore versus Bush), and the morale of surgeons (up versus down). On shuttle rides that week, I traded trauma stories with a general surgeon from Sleepy Eye, Minnesota, learned about Chinese hospitals from a British-accented vascular surgeon from Hong Kong, discussed autopsies with the University of Virginia's chairman of surgery, and got movie recommendations from a Cleveland surgical resident.

This is, I suppose, what the public relations professionals would call networking. But the word misses the essential hungriness of the doctors on those buses, and throughout the convention, for contact and belonging. We may have each had good practical reasons for coming here: the new ideas, the stuff to learn, the gizmos to try, the chasing of status, the break from the grind of unending responsibilities. But in the end, I came to think, there was also something more vital and, in a certain way, poignant drawing us in.

Doctors belong to an insular world—one of hemorrhages and lab tests and people sliced open. We are for the moment the healthy few who live among the sick. And it is easy to become alien to the experiences and sometimes the values of the rest of civilization. Ours is a world even our families do not grasp. This is, in certain respects, the experience of athletes and soldiers and professional musicians. Unlike them, however, we are not only removed, we are also alone. Once residency is over and you've settled in Sleepy Eye or the northern peninsula of Michigan or, for that matter, Manhattan, the slew of patients and isolation of practice take you away from anyone who really knows what it is like to cut a stomach cancer from a patient or lose her to a pneumonia afterward or answer the family's accusing questions or fight with insurers to get paid.

Once a year, however, there is a place full of people who do know. They are everywhere you look. They come and sit right next to you. The organizers call the convention its annual "Congress of Surgeons," and the words seem apt. We are, for a few days, with all the pluses and minuses it implies, our own nation of doctors.

When Good Doctors Go Bad

Hank Goodman is a former orthopedic surgeon. He is fifty-six years old and stands six feet one, with thick, tousled brown hair and out-size hands that you can easily imagine snapping a knee back into place. He is calm and confident, a man used to fixing bone. At one time, before his license was taken away, he was a highly respected and sought-after surgeon. "He could do some of the best, most brilliant work around," one of his orthopedic partners told me. When other doctors needed an orthopedist for family and friends, they called on him. For more than a decade, Goodman was among the busiest surgeons in his state. But somewhere along the way things started to go wrong. He began to cut corners, became sloppy. Patients were hurt, some terribly. Colleagues who had once admired him grew appalled. It was years, however, before he was stopped.

When people talk about bad doctors, they usually talk about the monsters. We hear about doctors like Harold Shipman, the physician from the North of England who was convicted of murdering fifteen patients with lethal doses of narcotics and is suspected of killing some three hundred in all. Or John Ronald Brown, a San Diego surgeon who, working without a license, bungled a series of sex-change operations and amputated the left leg of a perfectly healthy man, who then died of gangrene. Or James Burt, a notorious Ohio gynecologist who subjected hundreds of women, often after they had been anesthetized for other procedures, to a bizarre, disfiguring operation involving clitoral circumcision and vaginal "reshaping," which he called the Surgery of Love.

But the problem of bad doctors isn't the problem of these frightening aberrations. It is the problem of what you might call everyday bad doctors, doctors like Hank Goodman. In medicine, we all come to know such physicians: the illustrious cardiologist who has slowly gone senile and won't retire; the long-respected obstetrician with a drinking habit; the surgeon who has somehow lost his touch. On the one hand, strong evidence indicates that mistakes are not made primarily by this minority of doctors. Errors are too common and widespread to be explained so simply. On the other hand, problem doctors do exist. Even good doctors can go bad, and when they do, colleagues tend to be almost entirely unequipped to do anything about them.

Goodman and I talked over the course of a year. He sounded as baffled as anyone by what had become of him, but he agreed to tell his story so that others could learn from his experience. He even put me in touch with former colleagues and patients. His only request was that I not use his real name.

One case began on a hot August day in 1991. Goodman was at the hospital—a tentacled, modern, floodlit complex, with a towering red-brick building in the middle and many smaller facilities fanning out from it, all fed by an extensive network of outlying clinics and a nearby medical school. Situated off a long corridor on the ground floor of the main building were the operating rooms, with their white-tiled, wide-open spaces, the patients laid out, each under a canopy of lights, and teams of blue-clad people going about their business. In one of these rooms, Goodman finished an operation, pulled off his gown, and went over to a wall phone to respond to his messages while waiting for the room to be cleaned. One was from his physician assistant, at the office, half a block away. He wanted to talk to Goodman about Mrs. D.

Mrs. D was twenty-eight years old, a mother of two, and the wife of the business manager of a local auto-body shop. She had originally come to Goodman about a painless but persistent fluid swelling on her knee. He had advised surgery, and she had agreed to it. The week before, he had done an operation to remove the fluid. But now, the assistant reported, she was back; she felt feverish and ill, and her knee was intolerably painful. On examination, he told Goodman, the knee was red, hot, and tender. When he put a needle into the joint, foul-smelling pus came out. What should he do?

It was clear from this description that the woman was suffering from a disastrous infection, that she had to have the knee opened and drained as soon as possible. But Goodman was busy, and he never considered the idea. He didn't bring her into the hospital. He didn't go to see her. He didn't even have a colleague see her. Send her out on oral antibiotics, he said. The assistant expressed some doubt, to which Goodman responded, "Ah, she's just a whiner."

A week later, the patient came back, and Goodman finally drained her knee. But it was too late. The infection had consumed the cartilage. Her entire joint was destroyed. Later, she saw another orthopedist, but all he could do was fuse her knee solid to stop the constant pain of bone rubbing against bone.

When I spoke to her, she sounded remarkably philosophical. "I've adapted," she told me. With a solid knee, though, she said she can't run, can't bend down to pick up a child. She took several falls down the stairs of her split-level home, and she and her family had to move to a ranch-style house for safety's sake. She cannot sit on airplanes. In movie theaters, she has to sit sidewise on an aisle. Not long ago, she went to see a doctor about getting an artificial knee, but she was told that, because of the previous damage, it couldn't safely be done.

Every physician is capable of making a dumb, cavalier decision like Goodman's, but in his last few years of practice he made them over and over again. In one case, he put the wrong-size screw into a patient's broken ankle, and didn't notice that the screw had gone in too deep. When the patient complained of pain, Goodman refused to admit that anything needed to be done. In a similar case, he put a wrong-size screw into a broken elbow. The patient came back when the screw head had eroded through the skin. Goodman could easily have cut the screw to size, but he did nothing.

Another case involved an elderly man who'd come in with a broken hip. It looked as if he would need only a few pins to repair the fracture. In the operating room, however, the hip wouldn't come together properly. Goodman told me that he should have changed course and done a total hip replacement. But it had already been a strenuous day, and he couldn't endure the prospect of a longer operation. He made do with pins. The hip later fell apart and became infected. Each time the man came in, Goodman insisted there was nothing to be done. In time, the bone almost completely dissolved. Finally, the patient went to one of Goodman's colleagues for a second opinion. The colleague was horrified by what he found. "He ignored this patient's pleas for help," the surgeon told me. "He just wouldn't do anything. He literally wouldn't bring the patient into the hospital. He ignored the obvious on X rays. He could have killed this guy the way things were going."

For the last several years that Goodman was in practice, he was the defendant in a stream of malpractice suits, each of which he settled as quickly as he could. His botched cases became a staple of his department's Morbidity and Mortality conferences.

Sitting with him over breakfast in a corner of a downtown restaurant, I asked him how all this could have happened. Words seemed to elude him. "I don't know," he said faintly.

Goodman grew up in a small northwestern town, the second child of five in an electrical contractor's family, and neither he nor anyone else ever imagined that he might become a doctor. In college, a local state university, he was at first an aimless, mediocre student. Then one night he was up late drinking coffee, smoking cigarettes, and taking notes for a paper on a Henry James novel when it came to him: "I said to myself, 'You know, I think I'll go into medicine.'" It was not exactly an inspiration, he said. "I just came to a decision without much foundation I could ever see." A minister once told him that it sounded "more like a call than I ever got."

Goodman became a dedicated student, got into an excellent medical school, and headed for a career in surgery after graduation. After completing military duty as a general medical officer in the Air Force, he was accepted into one of the top orthopedics-residency programs in the country. He found the work deeply satisfying, despite the gruelling hours. He was good at it. People came in with intensely painful, disabling conditions—dislocated joints, fractured hips, limbs, spines—and he fixed them. "Those were the four best years of my life," he said. Afterward, he did some subspecialty training in hand surgery, and when he finished, in 1978, he had a wide range of choices for work. He ended up back in the Northwest, where he would spend the next fifteen years.

"When he came to the clinic here, we had three older, rusty and crusty orthopedic surgeons," a pediatrics colleague of his told me. "They were out of date and out of touch, and they weren't very nice to people. Then here comes this fellow, who's a sweetheart of a guy, more up to date, and he doesn't say no to anybody. You call him at eight o'clock at night with a kid who needs his hip tapped because of infection, and he'll come in and do it—and he's not even the one on call." He won a teaching award from his medical students. He attracted a phenomenal amount of business. He reveled in the job.

Sometime around 1990, however, things changed. With his skill and experience, Goodman knew better than most what needed to be done for Mrs. D, for the man with the shattered hip, and for many other patients, but he did not do it. What happened? All he could tell me was that everything seemed wrong those last few years. He used to enjoy being in the operating room, fixing people. After a while, though, it seemed that the only thing he thought about was getting through all his patients as quickly as possible.

Was money part of the problem? He made about two hundred thousand dollars a year at first, and the more patients he saw and the more cases he took the more money he made. Pushing himself, he found that he could make three hundred thousand dollars. Pushing himself even harder, until he was handling a dizzying number of cases, he made four hundred thousand dollars. He was far busier than any of his partners, and that fact increasingly became, in his mind, a key measure of his worth. He began to call himself, only half in jest, "The Producer." More than one colleague mentioned to me that he had become fixated on his status as the No. 1 booker.

His sense of himself as a professional also made him unwilling to turn people away. (He was, after all, the guy who never said no.) Whatever the cause, his caseload had clearly become overwhelming. He'd been working eighty, ninety, a hundred hours a week for well over a decade. He had a wife and three children—the children are grown now—but he didn't see much of them. His schedule was packed tight, and he needed absolute efficiency to get through it all. He'd begin with, say, a total hip replacement at 7:30 A.M. and try to finish in two hours or so. Then he'd pull off his gown, tear through the paperwork, and, as the room was being cleaned, stride out the main tower doors, into the sun, or snow, or rain, over to the outpatient-surgery unit, half a block away. He'd have another patient waiting on the table there—a simple case, maybe a knee arthroscopy or a carpal-tunnel release. Near the end, he'd signal a nurse to call ahead and have the next patient wheeled into the OR back in the main tower. He'd close skin on the second case and then bolt back for a third. He went back and forth all day. Yet, no matter what he did to keep up, unforeseen difficulties arose—a delay in getting a room ready, a new patient in the emergency room, an unexpected problem in an operation. Over time, he came to find the snags unbearable. That's undoubtedly when things became dangerous. Medicine requires the fortitude to take what comes: your schedule may be packed, the hour late, your child waiting for you to pick him up after swimming practice; but if a problem arises you have to do what is necessary. Time after time, Goodman failed to do so.

This sort of burnout is surprisingly common. Doctors are supposed to be tougher, steadier, better able to handle pressure than most. (Don't the rigors of medical training weed out the weak ones?) But the evidence suggests otherwise. Studies show, for example, that alcoholism is no less common among doctors than among other people. Doctors are more likely to become addicted to prescription narcotics and tranquilizers, presumably because we have such easy access to them. Some 32 percent of the general working-age population develops at least one serious mental disorder—such as major depression, mania, panic disorder, psychosis, or addiction—and there is no evidence that such disorders are any less common among doctors. And, of course, doctors become ill, old, and disaffected, or distracted by their own difficulties, and for these and similar reasons they falter in their care of patients. We'd all like to think of "problem doctors" as aberrations. The aberration may be a doctor who makes it through a forty-year career without at least a troubled year or two. Not everyone with "problems" is necessarily dangerous, of course. Nonetheless, estimates are that, at any given time, 3 to 5 percent of practicing physicians are actually unfit to see patients.

There's an official line about how the medical profession is supposed to deal with these physicians: colleagues are expected to join forces promptly to remove them from practice and report them to the medical-licensing authorities, who, in turn, are supposed to discipline them or expel them from the profession. It hardly ever happens that way. For no tight-knit community can function that way.

Marilynn Rosenthal, a sociologist at the University of Michigan, has examined how medical communities in the United States, Great Britain, and Sweden deal with problem physicians. She has gathered data on what happened in more than two hundred specific cases, ranging from a family physician with a barbiturate addiction to a fifty-three-year-old cardiac surgeon who continued operating despite permanent cerebral damage from a stroke. And nearly everywhere she looked she found the same thing. It was a matter of months, even years, before colleagues took effective action against a bad doctor, however dangerous his or her conduct might have been.

People have called this a conspiracy of silence, but Rosenthal did not find plotting so much as a sorry lack of it. In the communities she has observed, the dominant reaction was uncertainty, denial, and dithering, feckless intervention—very much like a family that won't face up to the fact that grandma needs to have her driver's license taken away. For one thing, not all problems are obvious: colleagues may suspect that Dr. So-and-So drinks too much or has become "too old," but certainty about such matters can remain elusive for a long time. Morever, even when problems *are* obvious, colleagues often find themselves unable to do anything decisive.

There are both honorable and dishonorable reasons for this. The dishonorable reason is that doing nothing is easy. It takes an enormous amount of work and self-assurance for colleagues to gather the evidence and the votes that are needed to suspend another doctor's privileges to practice. The honorable reason, and probably the main reason, is that no one really has the heart for it. When a skilled, decent, ordinarily conscientious colleague, whom you've known and worked with for years, starts popping Percodans, or becomes preoccupied with personal problems, and neglects the proper care of patients, you want to help, not destroy the doctor's career. There is no easy way to help, though. In private practice, there are no sabbaticals to offer, no leaves of absence, only disciplinary proceedings and public reports of misdeeds. As a consequence, when people try to help, they do it quietly, privately. Their intentions are good; the result usually isn't.

For a long time, Hank Goodman's colleagues tried to help him. Starting around 1990, they began to have suspicions. There was talk of the bizarre decisions, the dubious outcomes, the growing number of lawsuits. More and more, people felt the need to step in.

A few of the older physicians, each acting on his own, took him aside at one point or another. Rosenthal calls this the Terribly Quiet Chat. A partner would see Goodman at a cocktail party or just happen to drop by his home. He'd pull Goodman aside, ask how he was doing, tell him that people had concerns. Another took the tough-love approach: "I said to him straight out, 'I don't know what makes you tick. Your behavior is totally bizarre. The scary thing is I wouldn't let my family members go near you.'"

Sometimes this approach can work. I spoke to a retired department head at Harvard who had initiated more than a few Terribly Quiet Chats in his time. A senior physician can have forbidding moral authority in medicine. Many wayward doctors whom the department head confronted confessed to having troubles, and he did what he could to assist. He'd arrange to have them see a psychiatrist, or go to a drug rehab center, or retire. But some doctors didn't follow through. Others denied that anything was wrong. A few went so far as to mount small campaigns in their defense. They would have family members call him in outrage, loyal colleagues stop him in the hospital halls to say they'd never seen any wrongdoing, lawyers threaten to sue.

Goodman did listen to what people had to say. He nodded and confessed that he felt overworked, at times overwhelmed. He vowed to make changes, to accept fewer cases and stop rushing through them, to perform surgery as he knew it should be performed. He would walk away mortified, resolving to mend his ways. But in the end nothing changed.

As is often the case, the people who were in the best position to see how dangerous Goodman had become were in the worst position to do anything about it: junior physicians, nurses, ancillary staff. In such circumstances, the support staff will often take measures to protect patients. Nurses find themselves quietly directing patients to other doctors. Receptionists suddenly have trouble finding openings in a doctor's schedule. Senior surgical residents scrub in on junior-level operations to make sure a particular surgeon doesn't do anything harmful.

One of Goodman's physician assistants tried to take on this protective role. When he first began working with Goodman—helping to set fractures, following patients' progress, and assisting in the operating room—he revered the man. But he noticed when Goodman became erratic. "He'd run through forty patients in a day and not spend five minutes with them," the assistant told me. To avert problems in the clinic, he stayed late after hours, double-checking Goodman's decisions. "I was constantly following up with patients and changing what he did for them." In the operating room, he tried to make gentle suggestions. "Is that screw too long?" he might ask. "Does the alignment on that hip look right?" There were nonetheless mistakes and "a lot of unnecessary surgery," he said. When he could, he steered patients away from Goodman—"though without actually coming out and saying, 'I think he's crazy.'"

Matters can drift along this way for an unconscionably long time. But when someone has exhausted all reservoirs of goodwill—when the Terribly Quiet Chats are clearly going nowhere and there seems to be no end to the behind-the-scenes work colleagues have to do—the mood can change swiftly. The smallest matter can precipitate drastic action. With Goodman, it was skipping the mandatory weekly Morbidity and Mortality conferences, which he started to do in late 1993. As negligent as his patient care could be—he had become one of the hospital's most frequently sued doctors—people remained uncomfortable about judging him. When Goodman stopped attending M & Ms, however, his colleagues finally had a concrete violation to confront him with.

Various people warned him, with increasing sharpness, that he would be in serious trouble if he didn't start showing up at M & Ms. "But he ignored them all," a colleague of his told me. After a year of this, the hospital board put him on probation. Through it all, he was operating on more patients and generating ever more complications. Another whole year went by. Soon after Labor Day of 1995, the board and its lawyer finally sat him down at the end of a long conference table and told him that they were suspending his operating privileges and referring his conduct to the state medical board for investigation. He was fired.

Goodman had never let on to his family about his difficulties, and he didn't tell them that he'd lost his job. Each morning for weeks, he put on a suit and tie and went to his office, as if nothing had changed. He saw the last of his scheduled patients, and referred those who needed an operation to others. His practice dried up within a month. His wife sensed that something was wrong, and when she pressed him, he finally told her. She was floored, and frightened: she felt as if he were a stranger, an impostor. After that, he just stayed home in bed. He spoke to no one for days at a time.

Two months after his suspension, Goodman was notified of another malpractice suit, this one on behalf of a farmer's wife who had come to him with a severely arthritic shoulder. He had put in an artificial joint, but the repair failed. The lawsuit was the last straw. "I had nothing," he told me. "I had friends and family, yes, but no job." As with many doctors, his job was his identity.

In his basement den, he had a gun, a .44 Magnum that he had bought for a fishing trip to Alaska, to protect him against bears. He found the bullets for the gun and contemplated suicide. He knew how to do it so that his death would be instantaneous. He was, after all, a surgeon.

In 1998, I was at a medical conference near Palm Springs, skimming through the dense lecture schedule, when an unusual presentation caught my eye: "Two Hundred Physicians Reported for Disruptive Behavior," by Kent Neff, M.D. The lecture was in a small classroom away from the main lecture hall. At most, a few dozen people attended. Neff was fiftyish, trim, silver-haired, and earnest, and he turned out to have what must be the most closeted subspecialty in medicine: he was a psychiatrist specializing in doctors and other professionals with serious behavioral problems. In 1994, he told us, he had taken charge of a small program to help hospitals and medical groups with troubled doctors. Before long, they were sending him doctors from all over. To date, he'd seen more than two hundred and fifty, a remarkable wealth of experience, and he went through the data he'd collected like a CDC scientist analyzing an outbreak of tuberculosis.

What he found was unsurprising. The doctors were often not recognized to be dangerous until they had done considerable damage. They were rarely given a thorough evaluation for addiction, mental illness, or other typical afflictions. And, when problems were identified, the follow-through was abysmal. What impressed me was Neff's single-handed, quixotic attempt—he had no grants, no assistance from government agencies—to do something about this.

A few months after the lecture, I flew to Minneapolis to see Neff in action. His program was at Abbott Northwestern Hospital, near the city's Powderhorn district. When I arrived, I was directed to the fifth floor of a brick building discreetly off to one side of the main hospital complex. There I found a long, dimly lit hallway with closed, unmarked doors on both sides and beige, low-pile carpeting. It looked nothing like a hospital. A block-lettered sign read "Professional Assessment Program." Neff, in a tweed jacket and metal-rimmed glasses, came out of one of the doors and showed me around.

Each Sunday night, the physicians arrived here, suitcases in hand. They checked in down the hall and were shown to dormitory-style rooms where they would stay for four days and four nights. Three doctor-patients were staying during the week that I visited. They were permitted to come and go as they pleased, Neff assured me. Yet I knew that they were not quite free. In most cases, their hospitals had paid the program's fee of seven thousand dollars and told the doctors that if they wanted to keep their practices they had to go to Minneapolis.

The most striking aspect of the program, it seemed to me, was that Neff had actually persuaded medical organizations to send the doctors. He had done this, it seemed, by simply offering to help. For all their dithering, hospitals and clinics turned out to be eager for Neff's assistance. And they weren't the only ones. Before long, airlines began sending him pilots. Courts sent him judges. Companies sent him CEOs.

A small part of what Neff did was just meddle. He was like one of those doctors whom you consult about a coughing child, and who then tell you how to run your life. He'd take the doctors in hand, but he was not shy about telling organizations when they had let a problem fester too long. There are certain kinds of behavior—what he calls "behavioral sentinel events"—that should alert people that something may be seriously wrong with a person, he explains. For example, a surgeon throws scalpels in the OR, or a pilot bursts into uncontrolled rages in midflight. Yet, in case after case, such episodes are shrugged off. "He's a fine doctor," people will say, "but sometimes he has his moments."

Neff recognizes at least four types of behavioral sentinel events. There is persistent, poor anger control or abusive behavior. There is bizarre or erratic behavior. (He saw a doctor who could not get through the day without spending a couple of hours arranging and rearranging his desk. The doctor was found to have severe obsessive-compulsive disorder.) There is transgression of proper professional boundaries. (Neff once saw a family physician who was known to take young male patients out alone for dinner and, in one instance, on vacation with him. He turned out to have compulsive fantasies of sex with pubescent boys.) And there is the more familiar marker of incurring a disproportionate number of lawsuits or complaints (as Goodman had). Through his program, Neff has persuaded a substantial number of hospitals and clinics—and airlines and corporations—to take such events seriously. Many organizations have now specified, as a part of their contracts, that behavioral sentinel events could trigger an evaluation.

The essence of what he did, however, was simply to provide a patient consultation, the way a cardiologist might provide a consultation about someone's chest pains. He examined the person sent to him, performed some tests, and gave a formal opinion about what was going on, about whether the person could safely be kept on the job, and about how things might be turned around. Neff was willing to do what everyone else was extremely reluctant to do: to judge (or, as he prefers to say, to "assess") a fellow doctor. And he did it more thoroughly and dispassionately than a doctor's colleagues ever could.

Neff's first step with the three doctors seeing him the week I was there was to gather information. Starting on Monday morning, and throughout the next two days, he and four clinicians separately interviewed each of the doctors. They were made to tell their stories over and over again, half a dozen times or more, in order to break through their evasions and natural defensiveness, and to bring out the details. Before they arrived, Neff had also put together a thick dossier on each of them. And during the week he did not hesitate to call their colleagues back home in order to sort through the contradictions and ambiguities in their versions of events.

Neff's patients also underwent a full exam, including blood work, to make sure that no physical illness could account for any dangerous behavior. (One doctor, who was sent to Neff after several episodes of freezing in place in mid-operation, was found to have advanced Parkinson's disease.) They were given alcohol and drug testing. And they underwent psychological tests for everything from gambling addiction to paranoid schizophrenia.

On the last day, Neff assembled his team around a conference table in a drab little room to make their determinations. Meanwhile, the physicians waited in their rooms. The staff members spent about an hour reviewing the data in each case. Then, as a team, they made three separate decisions. First, they arrived at a diagnosis. Most doctors turned out to have a psychiatric illness—depression, bipolar disorder, drug or alcohol addiction, even outright psychosis. Almost without exception, the condition had never been diagnosed or treated. Others were simply struggling with stress, divorce, grief, illness, or the like. Next, the team decided whether the doctor was fit to return to practice. Neff showed me some typical reports. The judgment was always clear, unequivocal: "Due to his alcoholism, Dr. X cannot practice with reasonable skill and safety at this time." Last, they spelled out specific recommendations for the doctor to follow. For some doctors deemed fit to return to practice, they recommended certain precautions: ongoing random drug testing, formal monitoring by designated colleagues, special restrictions on the doctor's practice. For those found unfit, Neff and his team typically specified a minimum period of time away from their practice, a detailed course of treatment, and explicit procedures for reevaluation. At the end of the deliberations, Neff met in his office with each doctor and described the final report that would be sent to his hospital or clinic. "People are usually surprised," Neff told me. "Ninety percent find our recommendations more stringent than what they were expecting."

Neff reminded me more than once that his program provided only recommendations. But once he put his recommendations down on paper it was hard for hospitals and medical groups not to follow through and hold doctors to the plan. The virtue of Neff's approach was that once trouble occurred everything unfolded almost automatically: Minneapolis, evaluation, diagnosis, a plan. Colleagues no longer had to play judge and jury. And the troubled doctors got help. Neff and his team saved hundreds of careers from destruction—and possibly thousands of patients from harm.

Neff's was not the only program of its kind. In recent decades, medical societies here and abroad have established a number of programs to diagnose and treat "sick" physicians. But his was one of the very few independent programs and more systematic in its methods than just about any other.

Yet his program was shuttered a few months after my visit. Although it had attracted wide interest across the country and had grown rapidly, the Professional Assessment Program had struggled financially, never quite paying its own way. In the end, Neff was unable to persuade Abbott Northwestern Hospital to continue to subsidize it. He was, when we last spoke, seeking support to set up elsewhere.

But whether or not he succeeds, he has shown what can be done. The hard question—for doctors, and, even more, for their patients—is whether we can accept such an approach. Programs like Neff's cut a straightforward deal—maybe too straightforward. Physicians will turn in problematic colleagues—the ordinary, every-day bad doctors—only as long as the consequence is closer to diagnosis and treatment than to arrest and prosecution. And this requires that people be ready to view such doctors not as sociopaths but merely as struggling human beings. Neff's philosophy is, as he put it, "hard on behavior but soft on the person." People may actually prefer the world of don't ask, don't tell. Just ask yourself, could you abide by a system that rehabilitated drug-addicted anesthesiologists, cardiac surgeons with manic psychosis, or pediatricians with a thing for little girls if it meant catching more of them? Or, to put it another way, would you ever be ready to see Hank Goodman operate again?

Hank Goodman's life, and perhaps his career, was one of Kent Neff's saves. In mid-December of 1995, after pondering suicide, Goodman called Neff at his office. Goodman's lawyer had heard about the program and given him the number. Neff told him to come right away. Goodman made the trip the next day. They met for an hour, and at the end of the meeting Goodman remembers feeling that he could breathe again. Neff was direct and collegial and said that he could help him, that his life wasn't over. Goodman believed him.

He checked into the program the next week, paying for it himself. It was a difficult, at times confrontational, four days. He wasn't ready to admit all that he had done or to accept all that the members of Neff's team had found. The primary diagnosis was long-standing depression. Their conclusion was characteristically blunt: The doctor, they wrote, "is unable to practice safely now because of his major depression and will be unable to practice for an indefinite period of time." With adequate and prolonged treatment, the report said, "we would expect that he has the potential for a full return to practice." The particular diagnostic labels they gave him are probably less important than the intervention itself: the act of telling him, with institutional authority, that something was wrong with him, that he must not practice, and that he might be able to do so again one day.

At Neff's suggestion, Goodman checked into a psychiatric hospital. After that, a local psychiatrist and a supervising medical doctor were lined up to monitor him at home. He was put on Prozac, and then Effexor. He stuck with the program. "The first year, I didn't care if I lived or died," he told me. "The second year, I wanted to live but I didn't want to go to work. The third year, I wanted to go back to work." Eventually, his local psychiatrist, his internist, and Neff all agreed that he was ready. Largely on their advice, Goodman's state medical board has given him permission to return to practice, although with restrictions. At first, he would have to work no more than twenty hours a week and only under supervision. He had to see his psychiatrist and his medical doctor on a regular schedule. He could not operate for at least six months after returning to the clinic. Then he would be able to operate only as an assistant until a reevaluation determined that he could resume full privileges. He would also have to submit to random drug and alcohol tests.

But what practice would take him? His former partners wouldn't. "Too much baggage," he said. He came very close to securing a place in the rural lake town where he has a vacation home. It has a small hospital, visited by forty-five thousand people during the summer months, and no orthopedic surgeon. The doctors there were aware of his previous problems, but, having searched for an orthopedist for years, they approved his arrival. Still, it took almost a year for him to obtain malpractice insurance. And he thought it prudent to be cautious about returning to the stresses of a full-fledged practice. He decided to start off by doing physical examinations for an insurance company first.

Not long ago, I visited Goodman at his home, a modest brick ranch-style house full of dogs and cats and birds, tchotchkes in the living room, and, in a corner of the kitchen, a computer and a library of orthopedic journals and texts on CD-ROMs. He was dressed in a polo shirt and khakis, and he seemed loose, unhurried, almost indolent. Except for the time he spent with his family, and catching up on his field, he had little to occupy himself. His life could not have been further from that of a surgeon, but he felt the fire for the work coming back to him. I tried to picture him in surgeon's greens again—in an OR, with another assistant on the phone asking about a patient with an infected knee. Who could say how it would go?

We are all, whatever we do, in the hands of flawed human beings. The fact is hard to stare in the face. But it is inescapable. Every doctor has things he or she ought to know but has yet to learn, capacities of judgment that will fail, a strength of character that can break. Was I stronger than this man was now? More reliable? More conscientious? As aware and careful about my limitations? I wanted to think so—and perhaps I had to think so to do what I do day to day. But I could not know so. And neither could anyone else.

Goodman and I went out for a meal together in town and then for a drive. Coming upon his former hospital, gleaming and modern, I asked him if I could have a look around. He didn't have to come, I said. He had not been inside the building more than two or three times in the previous four years. After a momentary hesitation, he decided to join me. We walked in through the sliding automatic doors and down a polished white hallway. A sunny voice rang out, and I could see that he regretted having come in.

"Why, Dr. Goodman!" a smiling, matronly, white-haired woman said from behind the information desk. "I haven't seen you in years. Where have you been?"

Goodman stopped short. He opened his mouth to answer, but for a long moment nothing came out. "I retired," he said finally.

She tilted her head, obviously puzzled: Goodman looked robust and twenty years younger than she was. Then I saw her eyes sharpen as she began to catch on. "Well, I hope you're enjoying it," she said, recovering nicely.

He made an uncomfortable remark about all the fishing he was getting to do. We began to walk away. Then he stopped and spoke to her again. "I'll be back, though," he said.

Part II

Mystery

Full Moon Friday the Thirteenth

Jack Nicklaus would not play a round of golf without three pennies in his pocket. Michael Jordan always had to wear University of North Carolina boxer shorts under his Chicago Bulls uniform. And Duke Ellington would not play a show, or allow his band members to play a show, wearing anything yellow. For people who have to perform for a living, superstitions seem almost de rigueur. Baseball players, for example, are notoriously superstitious. Wade Boggs, the Boston Red Sox's former star third baseman, famously insisted on eating chicken before every game. Tommy Lasorda, on the other hand, when he was managing the Los Angeles Dodgers, always ate linguine—with either red clam sauce if his team was facing a right-handed pitcher, or white if up against a lefty. Even in this crowd, however, the New York Mets' pitcher Turk Wendell seems unusual. For luck during games, he used to wear an animal-fang necklace, refuse to wear socks, never step on the foul line, and brush his teeth between innings. When he signed his contract for the 1999 season, he insisted that his salary be $1,200,000.99. "Hey, I just like the number ninety-nine," he told the press.

I have yet to know, however, any doctors with such superstitions. Doctors tend to have a fierce commitment to the rational—surgeons especially. For one of the main satisfactions of science, and operating on people in particular, is the success of logical planning and thinking. If there is a credo in practical medicine, it is that the important thing is to be sensible. And we who are in it are usually uncomfortable, if not outright contemptuous, of the mystical. At the most, you might find a surgeon with a favorite pair of operating shoes or a quirky way of dressing a wound after closing up. And even then we are always careful to account for our idiosyncracies with at least a plausible-sounding explanation: "Other shoes aren't as comfortable," the surgeon might say, or, "That dressing tape causes blisters" (though no one else seems to have trouble with it). As a rule, you will not find doctors saying that, actually, we just think a thing is unlucky.

So it struck me as odd to find, one afternoon when I and my fellow surgical residents sat around a table divvying up the next month's schedule of nights on emergency room duty, that no one was volunteering to take Friday the thirteenth. We were taking turns making picks, and for the first few rounds, everything seemed normal. We left all the Fridays alone, weekend nights not being popular. But as the nights remaining dwindled to just a few, it became apparent that that one Friday was being conspicuously bypassed. C'mon, I thought, this is ridiculous. So when my turn came up again, I put my name down for duty that night. "Rest up," one resident said. "You're going to be in for a busy night." I laughed and dismissed the idea.

Looking at my calendar a few days later, however, I noticed that the moon would also be full that Friday night. Then someone mentioned that a lunar eclipse would be occurring then, too. And for a moment—only a moment, mind you—I felt my confidence slip. Perhaps I really would be in for a miserable night, I began to think. But being a sober and well-trained doctor, I did not let myself succumb to such thoughts so easily. Surely, I thought, the evidence is against such preposterousness. And then, just to confirm it, I went to the library to check.

I managed to find exactly one scientific study assessing whether or not luck actually does go bad on Friday the thirteenth. (I'm not sure which is more surprising: that people have in fact researched this question, or that I could only find one such example. This is, after all, a world with studies on almost anything you could think of. Once, poking around the library, I even found a report on how saliva distributes around the mouth when chewing gum.) The 1993 study, published in the *British Medical Journal*, compared hospital admissions for traffic accidents on a Friday the thirteenth with those on a Friday the sixth in a community outside London. Despite a lower highway traffic volume on the thirteenth than on the sixth, admissions for traffic accident victims increased 52 percent on the thirteenth. "Friday the thirteenth is unlucky for some," the authors concluded. "Staying at home is recommended." How you escape the bad luck at home they didn't explain.

Still, I told myself, you really can't make much of one study of one Friday the thirteenth in one town. Random variation could easily have accounted for the increase in crashes. You would need to see consistently bad results across a number of studies to be convinced. And that has yet to be shown.

By contrast, one thing that has been shown is that human beings commonly imagine patterns (whether good or bad) where really there are none. It's just how our brains work. Even totally random patterns will often appear non-random to us. The statistician William Feller described one now classic example. During the Germans' intensive bombing of South London in the Second World War, a few areas were hit many times over while some others were not hit at all. The places that were not hit seemed to have been deliberately spared, and people concluded that those places were where the Germans had their spies. When Feller analyzed the statistics of the bomb hits, however, he found that the distribution was purely random.

This propensity to see nonexistent patterns has been called the Texas-sharpshooter fallacy. Like a Texas sharpshooter who shoots at the side of a barn and then draws a bull's-eye around the bullet holes, we tend to notice unusual occurrences first—four bad things happening on one day, for example—and then define a pattern around them. It seems to me we could just as well have feared Thursday the thirteenth, or Friday the fifth, as Friday the thirteenth. Nonetheless, phobia about Friday the thirteenth is widespread. Based on surveys, Donald Dossey, a North Carolina behavioral scientist, estimates that between seventeen million and twenty-one million Americans suffer mild to severe anxiety or change their activities because of *paraskevidekatriaphobia* (which is Greek for "fear of Friday the thirteenth"). They perform rituals before leaving the house, call in sick to work, or postpone flights or major purchases, causing businesses to lose seven hundred and fifty million dollars annually.

Superstitions about the moon appear to be taken even more seriously. A 1995 poll found that 43 percent of Americans believed that the moon alters individual behavior. And, interestingly, mental health professionals were more likely to believe it than people in other lines of work. The full moon has been thought to be linked to madness for centuries—hence the term "lunatic"—and in disparate civilizations across the world. Certainly, the idea of lunar human cycles seems more plausible than a Friday-the-thirteenth effect. Scientists once dismissed the idea of biological cycles, but now widely accept that season can affect mood and behavior and that we all have "circadian rhythms" in which time of day affects body temperature, alertness, memory, and mood.

In a computer search, I managed to find some one hundred studies that attempted to identify "circalunidian" cycles. The most intriguing one I looked up was a five-year study of self-poisoning at a hospital in New South Wales, Australia, published in the *Medical Journal of Australia*. From 1988 to 1993, the hospital admitted 2,215 patients for overdosing on drugs or poisoning themselves with toxic substances. The researchers checked to see whether peaks in such events occurred not just according to the phase of the moon but also according to one's zodiac sign or numerological readings (as "calculated according to the formulas contained in *Zolar's Encyclopedia of Ancient and Forbidden Knowledge,*" the authors reported). To no one's surprise, self-poisoning rates were not affected by whether a patient was born a Virgo or a Libra. Nor did Zolar's "Name Number," "Month Number," or "Birth Path Number" for a person make any difference. However, women (but not men) were about 25 percent *less* likely to overdose around the time of a full moon than around a new moon.

Strangely enough, this decrease in self-poisonings actually correlated with the results of other studies. If any link between psychology and the full moon exists, it would seem to be protective. The authors of a 1996 study of ten years of suicides in the Dordogne region of France concluded, in charmingly ungrammatical English, that "the French dies less in Full Moon, and more in New Moon period." Studies in Cuyahoga County, Ohio, and Dade County, Florida, also found a drop in suicides at the full moon. These studies didn't quite clinch the full moon's happy effect, however. Far more studies failed to find any lunar correlation with suicide.

As for other forms of craziness, the moon seems to play no role. Researchers have reviewed logs for calls to police stations, consultations to psychiatrists, homicides, and other records of our daily burden of madness—including, I noticed, emergency room visits. They found no consistent relationship, one way or another, with the moon.

Reassured by this, I was finally able to leave the library convinced that neither the full moon nor the inauspicious date threatened my night on call. A couple of weeks later the appointed evening arrived. I walked into the ER at 6 P.M. sharp to take over from the daytime resident. To my dismay, he was already swamped with patients for me to see. Then, just as soon as I began to get caught up, a fresh trauma came in—a pale and bloodied twenty-eight-year-old knocked unconscious in a high-speed head-on collision. The police and paramedics said he had been stalking his girlfriend with a gun in hand. The cops then arrived and he fled in his car, leading them on a chase that ended in the massive crash.

The rest of the night went no better. I was, as we say, "slammed" — running hard, unable to get two minutes to sit down, hardly able to keep the patients straight.

"It's full moon Friday the thirteenth," a nurse explained.

I was about to say that, actually, the studies show no connection. But my pager went off before I could get the words out of my mouth. I had a new trauma coming in.

The Pain Perplex

Every pain has a story, and the story of Rowland Scott Quinlan's goes back to an accident that happened years ago, when he was fifty-six. A Boston architect and avid sailor with a shock of white hair and a predilection for bow ties and Dutch cigarillos, Quinlan headed a thriving Beacon Street firm in his name and had designed such buildings as the University of Massachusetts Medical School. Then, in March of 1988, he fell off a plank at the construction site of one of his commissions—a pavilion at the Franklin Park Zoo. His back was fine, but he dislocated and fractured his left shoulder, and it required several operations. In the fall, he returned to his drafting table, and there he was hit by a spasm of pain like a writhing snake in his back. The attacks recurred, and although at first he tried to ignore them, they soon became unbearable. More than once, while he was standing with a client the back pain suddenly burst forth and it was all he could do to keep from crying out while the client caught him and helped him to a seat or to the floor. Sitting in a restaurant with a colleague, he was overcome by pain so severe that he vomited right there at the table. Soon he wasn't able to work more than two or three hours a day, and he had to give up the firm to his partners.

Quinlan's orthopedist had taken numerous X rays. They revealed little—perhaps a bit of arthritis, but nothing out of the ordinary. So Quinlan was sent to a pain specialist, who injected a long-needle syringe full of steroids and local anesthetic into his spine. The first few of these epidural injections worked for days, sometimes weeks, but subsequent shots provided steadily diminishing relief, until they didn't work at all.

I had seen his CT scans along with a sheaf of other tests and medical images. Nothing in them would have led me to expect the severity of his back pain: there was no fracture, no tumor, no infection, not even a sign of arthritic inflammation. The vertebrae were aligned perfectly, like checkers in a stack. None of the soft gel-like disks that sit like cushions between the vertebrae had ruptured. In the lower back, the lumbar spine, two disks bulged a bit, but that is common in men of his age, and the bulges didn't seem to be pressing against any nerves. Even an intern could see that there was no cause for operating on this back.

When doctors encounter a patient who has chronic pain without physical findings to account for it—and such patients are exceedingly common—we tend to be dismissive. We believe the world to be decipherable and logical, to come with problems we can see or feel or at least measure with some machine. So a pain like Quinlan's, we're apt to conclude, is all in the head: not a physical pain but a different, somehow less real, "mental" pain. In fact, Quinlan's orthopedist recommended that he see a psychiatrist as well as a physical therapist.

When I visited Quinlan at his home, in a seaside town outside Boston, I found him at what turned out to be his usual perch: a worktable in the kitchen facing a wall-length window with a view of a small garden. Blueprints of unfinished projects were curled up in rolls on the table. A telephone headset lay to one side. A dozen different kinds of drawing pens, along with small rulers and a protractor, sat in a holder. He grimaced as he rose to greet me. I thought about his thorough medical workup and those clean images of his spine: Was he faking it?

When I asked him, he smiled wanly, and told me he sometimes wondered that himself. "I've got it pretty cushy here," he said. Quinlan has handicap license plates, financial security, and none of the pressures of running a business, and if he doesn't want to do something he merely has to say his back is killing him. But, despite a patch on his arm that infuses high doses of the narcotic fentanyl through his skin twenty-four hours a day, he can't do even the simplest thing—stand in a line, walk up stairs, or even sleep more than four hours at a stretch—without the acute sensation that, as he puts it, "someone is wringing out a muscle in my back."

I asked his wife, a tall woman several years younger than him with fine features and sad eyes, if she ever thought he fakes the pain. She told me that day in and day out for a decade now she has seen the pain and lived with the increasing limits it places on his life and hers. She has seen the pain defeat him in ways that she knows he is too proud to fake. He'll try to carry the groceries, and then, shamefaced, have to hand them back a few moments later. Though he loves movies, they have not been to the cinema in years. There have been times when the pain of movement has been so severe that he has soiled his pants rather than make his way to the bathroom.

Yet there are aspects of the pain that puzzle her and make her wonder whether it is in some respects in his head. She notices that when he is anxious or irritable, the pain is worse, and that when he is in a good mood or is simply distracted, the pain can disappear. He has bouts of depression which seem to bring on terrible spasms almost regardless of what he is doing physically. Like his physicians, she wonders how a pain can be so incapacitating yet arise from no identifiable physical abnormality. And what about the circumstances that tend to bring on an attack—a mood, a thought, sometimes nothing at all? These traits strike her as unusual, as needing explanation. But the disturbing truth is that Roland Scott Quinlan isn't unusual. Among chronic pain sufferers, his case is altogether typical.

Dr. Edgar Ross, an anesthesiologist in his forties, is the director of the chronic-pain treatment center at Brigham and Women's Hospital in Boston, where Quinlan is seen. Patients come to Dr. Ross with every imaginable kind of pain: back pain, neck pain, arthritic pain, total-body pain, neuropathic pain, AIDS-related pain, pelvic pain, chronic headaches, cancer pain, phantom-limb pain. Often, they have already seen numerous doctors and tried multiple therapies, including surgery, to no avail.

The center's waiting room looks like any other doctor's office. It has the flat blue carpet, the dated magazines, the row of expressionless patients sitting silently against the wall. A glass case displays thank-you letters. But when I visited Dr. Ross recently I noticed that the letters were not quite the typical testimonials that doctors like to put up. These patients did not thank the doctors for a cure. They thanked the doctors merely for taking their pain seriously—for believing in it. The truth is that doctors like me are grateful to the pain specialists, too. Though we want to be neutral in our feelings toward patients, we'll admit among ourselves that chronic-pain patients are a source of frustration and annoyance: presenting a malady we can neither explain nor alleviate, they shake our claims to competence and authority. We're all too happy to have someone like Dr. Ross to take these patients off our hands.

Ross led me into his office. Soft-spoken and unhurried, he has a soothing demeanor that fits perfectly with his line of work. Quinlan's kind of problem, he told me, is the one he sees most frequently. Chronic back pain is now second only to the common cold as a cause of lost work time, and it accounts for some 40 percent of workers' compensation payments. In fact, there is a virtual epidemic of back pain in this country today, and nobody can explain why. By convention, we think of it as a mechanical problem, the result of misplaced stress on the spine. We therefore have had some sixty years of workplace programs, and now there are even "back schools," which teach the "correct way to lift," among other things. Despite the fact that the number of people who engage in manual labor has steadily declined, however, more people have chronic back pain than have ever had it before.

The mechanical explanation is almost certainly wrong, Ross noted. It's true that lifting something the wrong way can cause a muscle pull or a slipped disk. But that sort of strain occurs in almost everyone at some time, and in most people it never becomes a persistent problem. Scores of studies have looked for physical factors that can predict which acute back injuries will evolve into chronic back pain, but they haven't found any. For instance, doctors used to assume that damaged disks were associated with pain, but recent findings have not borne this out. Spinal MRI scans show that most people without back pain have disk bulges. Conversely, a large percentage of patients with chronic back pain, like Quinlan, are found to have no structural lesion. And even among those with abnormalities there is no relation between the severity of the pain and the severity of the abnormalities.

If the condition of your back doesn't predict whether you'll get chronic back pain, what does? Well, it's the mundane stuff that neither doctors nor patients much like to consider. Studies point to such "inorganic" factors as loneliness, involvement in litigation, receipt of workers' compensation, and job dissatisfaction. Consider, for example, the epidemic of back pain in the medical profession itself. Disability insurers once saw doctors as ideal customers. Nothing stopped doctors from working—not years of stooping over operating tables, not arthritis, not even old age. Insurers used to try to outbid one another with cheap rates and generous benefits to attract their business. In the last few years, however, the number of doctors with disabling back or neck pain has risen dramatically. Needless to say, doctors aren't suddenly being required to carry heavy packages around. But one known risk factor has been identified: with the growing role of managed care, job satisfaction in the medical profession has plunged.

The explanation of pain that has dominated much of medical history originated with René Descartes, more than three centuries ago. Descartes proposed that pain is a purely physical phenomenon—that tissue injury stimulates specific nerves that transmit an impulse to the brain, causing the mind to perceive pain. The phenomenon, he said, is like pulling on a rope to ring a bell in the brain. It is hard to overstate how ingrained this account has become. Twentieth-century research on pain has been devoted largely to the search for and discovery of pain-specific nerve fibers (now named A-delta and C fibers) and pathways. In everyday medicine, doctors see pain in Cartesian terms—as a physical process, a sign of tissue injury. We look for a ruptured disk, a fracture, an infection, or a tumor, and we try to fix what's wrong.

The limitations of this mechanistic explanation, however, have been apparent for some time. During the Second World War, for example, Lieutenant Colonel Henry K. Beecher conducted a classic study of men with serious battlefield injuries. In the Cartesian view, the degree of injury ought to determine the degree of pain, rather like a dial controlling volume. Yet 58 percent of the men—men with compound fractures, gunshot wounds, torn limbs—reported only slight pain or no pain at all. Just 27 percent of the men felt enough pain to request pain medication, although such wounds routinely require narcotics in civilians. Clearly, something that was going on in their minds—Beecher thought they were overjoyed to have escaped alive from the battlefield—counteracted the signals sent by their injuries. Pain was becoming recognized as far more complex than a one-way transmission from injury to "ouch."

In 1965, the Canadian psychologist Ronald Melzack and the British physiologist Patrick Wall proposed that the Cartesian model be replaced with what they called the Gate-Control Theory of Pain.

Melzack and Wall argued that before pain signals reach the brain they must first go through a gating mechanism in the spinal cord, which could ratchet them up or down. In some cases, this hypothetical gate could simply stop pain impulses from getting to the brain. In fact, researchers soon identified a gate for pain in a portion of the spinal cord called the dorsal horn. The theory explained such ordinary puzzles as why rubbing a painful foot makes it feel better. (The rubbing sends signals to the dorsal horn that close the gate to nearby pain impulses.)

Melzack and Wall's most startling suggestion was that what controlled the gate was not just signals from sensory nerves but also emotions and other "output" from the brain. They were saying that pulling on the rope need not make the bell ring. The bell itself—the mind—could stop it. Their theory prompted a great deal of research into how factors such as mood, gender, and beliefs influence the experience of pain. In one study, for example, researchers measured pain threshold and tolerance levels in fifty-two dancers from a British ballet company and fifty-three university students using a standard method called the cold-pressor test. The test is ingeniously simple. (I tried it at home myself.) After immersing your hand in body-temperature water for two minutes to establish a baseline condition, you dunk your hand in a bowl of ice water and start a clock running. You mark the time when it begins to hurt: that is your pain threshold. Then you mark the time when it hurts too much to keep your hand in the water: that is your pain tolerance. The test is always stopped at a hundred and twenty seconds, to prevent injury.

The results were striking. On average, female students reported pain at sixteen seconds and pulled their hands out of the ice water at thirty-seven seconds. Female dancers went almost three times as long on both counts. Men in both groups had a higher threshold and tolerance for pain—as expected, since studies show women to be more sensitive than men to pain, except during the last few weeks of pregnancy—but the difference between male dancers and male nondancers was nearly as large. What explains the difference?

Probably it has something to do with the psychology of ballet dancers—a group distinguished by self-discipline, physical fitness, and competitiveness, as well as by a high rate of chronic injury. Their driven personalities and competitive culture evidently inure them to pain: that's why they are able to perform through sprains and stress fractures, and why half of all dancers develop long-term injuries. (Similar to other nondancing males, I started to feel pain at around twenty-five seconds; but I had no trouble keeping my hand in for the whole hundred and twenty seconds. I will let others speculate on what this says about the submissiveness inculcated in surgical residents.)

Other studies along these lines have shown that extroverts have greater pain tolerance than introverts, that drug abusers have low pain tolerance and thresholds, and that, with training, one can diminish one's sensitivity to pain. There is also striking evidence that very simple kinds of mental suggestion can have powerful effects on pain. In one study of five hundred patients undergoing dental procedures, those who were given a placebo injection and reassured that it would relieve their pain had the least discomfort—not only less than the patients who got a placebo and were told nothing but also less than the patients who got a real anesthetic without any reassuring comment that it would work. Today, it is abundantly evident that the brain is actively involved in the experience of pain, and is no mere bell on a string. Today, every medical textbook teaches the Gate-Control Theory as fact. There's a problem with it, though. It doesn't explain people like Roland Scott Quinlan.

Gate-Control Theory accepts Descartes's view that what you feel as pain is a signal from tissue injury transmitted by nerves to the brain, and it adds the notion that the brain controls a gateway for such an injury signal. But in the case of Quinlan's chronic back pain, where is the injury? Or take something like phantom-limb pain. After amputation of a limb, most people suffer a period of constant, intractable burning or cramping that feels exactly as if the limb were still there. Without a limb, however, there are no nerve impulses for the gate to control. So where does the pain come from? The rope and clapper are gone, but the bell can still ring.

One spring day in 1994, Dr. Frederick Lenz, a neurosurgeon at the Johns Hopkins Hospital, brought to his operating table a patient suffering from severe hand tremors. The patient, whom I'll call Mark Taylor, was only thirty-six, but over the years his hands had come to shake so violently that the simplest of tasks—writing, buttoning his shirt, drinking from a glass, or typing on his keyboard at his job as a purchasing agent—grew absurdly difficult. Medications failed, and he lost jobs more than once because of his difficulties. Desperate for a return to a normal life, he agreed to a delicate procedure: brain surgery that would destroy cells in a small structure called the thalamus, which was already known to contribute to such excessive stimulation of the hands.

Taylor had another big problem, though: for seventeen years, he had struggled with a severe panic disorder. At least once a week, while he was working at his computer terminal or was at home in the kitchen feeding a child, he would suddenly be overcome by severe chest pains, as if he were having a heart attack. His heart would pound, his ears would ring; he would grow short of breath and would have an overwhelming urge to escape. Nevertheless, a psychologist Lenz consulted assured him that the disorder was unlikely to hinder the operation.

Initially, Lenz says, everything went as he had expected. He injected a local anesthetic—the operation is done with the patient awake—and burred a small opening in the top of Taylor's skull. Then he cautiously inserted a long, thin electrical probe deep inside, right down into the thalamus. Lenz talked to Taylor the whole time, asking him to stick out his tongue, to move a hand, to do any of a dozen other tasks that showed he was all right. The danger in this type of surgery is that it might destroy the wrong cells: the thalamic cells involved in tremor lie just fractions of a millimeter away from cells that are essential for sensation and motor activity. So before cauterizing with a second, larger probe, the surgeon had to find the right cells by stimulating them with a gentle electric pulse. The probe was in a portion of Taylor's thalamus that Lenz labeled Site 19, and he zapped it with low voltage. He had been here a thousand times before, and typically, he told me, zapping the site makes people feel a prickle in the forearm. Sure enough, this is what Taylor felt. Lenz then zapped an adjacent area he labeled Site 23, where stimulation generally produces a mild and very ordinary tingling in the chest. This time, however, Taylor felt an unexpectedly far more harsh pain—in fact, the exact chest pain of his panic attacks, along with the suffocation and instant sense of doom that always accompanied them. It made him cry out and nearly leap off the table. When Lenz stopped the stimulation, however, the sensation disappeared, and Taylor became instantly calm again. Puzzled, Lenz zapped Site 23 once more, and found that doing so produced the same effect again. He stopped, apologized to Taylor for the discomfort, and went on to locate the cells controlling his tremor and to cauterize them. The operation was a success.

Yet even as Lenz completed the procedure, his mind was racing. Only once before had he seen anything like this kind of effect. It was in a sixty-nine-year-old woman with a long history of difficult-to-manage anginal pain that came on not only with strenuous activity but even with mild physical exertion that wouldn't be expected to stress her heart. Performing a similar operation on her, Lenz found that stimulating the microscopic section of her brain that usually triggered mild chest tingling had instead, as with Taylor, brought on her more severe and familiar chest pain—a sensation she described as "deep, frightful, squeezing." The implications might have easily been lost, but Lenz had spent many years researching pain and realized that he had witnessed an important and telling effect. As he later noted in a report published in the journal *Nature Medicine*, the response in these two patients was wildly out of proportion to the stimulus. What in most people produces no more than a tingle was torture to them. Areas of the brain governing ordinary sensations appeared to have become abnormally sensitized—set to fire in response to perfectly harmless stimuli. In the woman's case, her chest pain had begun as a signal of her heart disease but now appeared in circumstances that did not reflect anything like an impending heart attack. Even more oddly, in Taylor's case, the pain had not begun with any such bodily damage, but with his panic disorder, which is understood to be a psychological condition. Lenz's findings suggest that, in fact, all pain is "in the head"—and further that sometimes, as with Mark Taylor or perhaps Roland Scott Quinlan, no physical injury of any kind is needed to make the pain system go haywire.

This is the newest theory of pain. Its leading proponent is, once again, Melzack, who abandoned Gate-Control Theory in the late 1980s and began telling incredulous audiences to revise their understanding of pain once again. Given the evidence, he now says, we should stop thinking that pain or any other sensation is a signal passively "felt" in the brain. Yes, injury produces nerve signals that travel through a spinal-cord gate, but it is the brain that generates the pain experience, and it can do so even in the absence of external stimuli. If a mad scientist reduced you to nothing but a brain in a jar, Melzack says, you could still feel pain—indeed, you could have the full range of sensory experience.

According to the new theory, pain and other sensations are conceived as "neuromodules" in the brain—something akin to individual computer programs on a hard drive, or to tracks on a compact disc. When you feel pain, it's your brain running a neuromodule that produces the pain experience, as if someone pressed the PLAY button on a CD player. And a great many things can press the button (besides a neurosurgeon zapping the right neuron with low DC voltage). The way Melzack explains it, a pain neuromodule is not a discrete anatomical entity but a network, linking components from virtually every region of the brain. Input is gathered from sensory nerves, memory, mood, and other centers, like members of some committee in charge of whether the music will play. If the signals reach a certain threshold, they trigger the neuromodule. And then what plays is no one-note melody. Pain is a symphony—a complex response that includes not just a distinct sensation but also motor activity, a change in emotion, a focusing of attention, a brand-new memory.

Suddenly, a simple toe-stubbing no longer seems so simple. In this view, the signal from the toe still has to make it through the spinal-cord gate, but thereafter it joins a lot of other signals in the brain—from memories, anticipation, mood, distractions. Altogether, they may combine to activate a toe-pain neuromodule. In some people, however, the physical stimulus may be canceled out and the stubbed toe hardly noticed. There's nothing surprising here so far. But now we can imagine—and this is the most radical implication of Melzack's ideas—that the same neuromodule can go off, generating genuine toe pain, without a toe's having been stubbed at all. The neuromodule could—like Site 23 in Mark Taylor's brain—become primed like a hair trigger. Then virtually anything could set it off: a touch, a stab of fear, a sudden frustration, a mere memory.

The new theory about the psychology of pain has, almost perversely, helped give direction to the pharmacology of pain. For pharmacologists, the Holy Grail of chronic-pain treatment is a pill that would be more effective than morphine but lack its side effects, such as dependence, sedation, and motor impairment. If an overactive neuronal system is the problem, then what one needs is a drug that will damp it down. That's why, in what a decade ago might have seemed a strange development, pain specialists increasingly prescribe anti-epileptic drugs, like carbamazepine and gabapentin, for their most difficult-to-treat patients. After all, that's what these drugs do: they tune brain cells to modulate their excitability. So far, these kinds of drugs work only for some people—Quinlan has been on gabapentin for more than six months without much effect—but drug companies are hard at work on a new generation of similar "neuro-stabilizing" compounds.

Neurex, for example, a small Silicon Valley biotechnology company (now called Elan Pharmaceuticals), not long ago designed a pain drug from the venom of the Conus sea snail following such thinking. Venoms are, needless to say, biologically potent, and, unlike most of the proteins from nature that scientists have tried to use as drugs, they evade the body's mechanisms for breaking proteins down. The trick is to tame the venom, to modify it so it is medically useful. The Conus venom was known to kill by blocking specific pathways in the brain that are necessary in order for neurons to fire. With a few alterations, however, Neurex scientists created Ziconotide, a drug that only slightly inhibits those pathways. Instead of shutting brain cells down, it seems to merely mute their excitability. In initial clinical trials, Ziconotide effectively controlled chronic pain from cancer and from AIDS. Another new generation analgesic in development is Abbott Laboratories' ABT-594, a compound related to a poison secreted by an Ecuadorian frog, *Epibpedobates tricolor*. In animal experiments that were published in the journal *Science*, ABT-594 proved to be as much as fifty times as potent as morphine in relieving pain. Companies have other pain drugs in the pipeline, too, including a class of drugs known as NMDA antagonists, which also work by reducing neuronal excitability. One of these could turn out to be the painkiller that Quinlan and patients like him are looking for.

At best, however, these drugs represent only a halfway solution. The fundamental problem for research is how to stop the pain system in such patients from going haywire in the first place. The stories that people tell of their chronic pain typically start with an initial injury. So, historically, we have tried to prevent chronic pain by preventing acute strains. A whole ergonomics industry has developed around this idea. Yet the lesson from Ross's pain clinic and Lenz's operating table is that the antecedents of pain lie elsewhere than in the muscle and bone of patients. In fact, some forms of chronic pain behave astonishingly like social epidemics.

In Australia during the early 1980s, workers—particularly keyboard operators—experienced a sudden outbreak of disabling arm pain, which doctors labeled "repetition strain injury," or RSI. This was not a mild case of writer's cramp but a matter of severe pain, which started with minor discomfort during typing or other repetitive work and progressed to invalidism. The average time that a sufferer lost from work was seventy-four days. As with chronic back pain, no consistent physical abnormalities or effective treatment could be found, yet the arm pain spread like a contagion. It had hardly existed before 1981, but by its peak, in 1985, enormous numbers of workers were affected. In two Australian states, RSI disabled as much as 30 percent of the workforce in some industries; at the same time there were pockets of workers who were almost entirely unaffected. Clusters appeared even within a single organization. At Telecom Australia, for example, the incidence of RSI among telephone operators in a single city varied widely between departments. Nor could investigators find any connection between RSI and the physical circumstances of the workers—the actual repetitiveness of their jobs or the ergonomics of their equipment. Then, as suddenly as it had begun, the epidemic crashed. By 1987, it was essentially over. In the late 1990s, Australian researchers were complaining that they couldn't find enough RSI patients to study.

Chronic back pain has been with us for so long that it is hard conceptually—and even politically—to step back and recognize its social etiology, let alone figure out how cultural factors make an individual's pain system go awry. The Australian pain epidemic demonstrates the power of those factors to cause genuine, disabling pain on a national scale, and yet our knowledge of these causes and how to control them is meager. We know from a variety of studies that social-support networks—a happy marriage and satisfying employment, say—protect against disabling back pain. We know, statistically speaking, that being given certain diagnostic labels and being provided disability pay (and thus a kind of official recognition and validation) can perpetuate chronic pain. In Australia, for example, many researchers believe that two major factors that sparked the epidemic were the coining of RSI as a diagnostic label and early action by the government to insure compensation for the syndrome as a work-related disability. When the diagnosis fell out of favor with physicians, and disability coverage became harder to get, the incidence of the symptoms associated with the disorder plummeted. It also appeared that initial publicity about the possible portents of arm pain and concerted campaigns in some places to increase the reporting of arm pains or to institute ergonomic changes only contributed to the epidemic. More recently, in the United States, a debate has erupted over the origins of a similar workplace epidemic, called, variously, repetitive-stress injury, repetitive-motion disorder, and—in the currently favored nomenclature—cumulative-trauma disorder. Once again, the salient risk factors seem to be social rather than physical.

Back and arm pain are not unique in having nonphysical causes. Studies have shown that social conditions play a dominant role in many chronic-pain syndromes, including chronic pelvic pain, temporomandibular-joint disorder, and chronic tension headache, to name just a few. Again, none of this should be taken to mean that people are faking it. As Melzack's account suggests, pain that doesn't arise from physical injury is no less real than pain that does—in the brain it is precisely the same. And so a compassionate approach toward chronic pain means investigating its social coordinates, not just its physical ones. For the solution to chronic pain may lie more in what goes on around us than in what is going on inside us. Of all the implications of the new theory of pain, this one seems to be the oddest and the most far-reaching: it has made pain political.

A Queasy Feeling

In the beginning, the nausea didn't seem anything to worry about. Amy Fitzpatrick was eight weeks pregnant—with twins, as an ultrasound had revealed—and, having watched her sister and her friends go through their pregnancies, she understood that nausea was simply part of the deal. Her first episode was certainly inconvenient, though. She was on New York City's F.D.R. Drive, piloting her Honda Civic to work through the frantic rush of morning traffic. Speeding along at fifty miles per hour, she realized that she was about to throw up.

Fitzpatrick was twenty-nine years old, tall, with long, thick black hair set against pale Irish skin and a dimpled, almost teenage face that sometimes made it hard for people to take her seriously, despite her Wharton M.B.A. She lived in Manhattan, where her husband was an investment banker, and she commuted to Manhasset, on Long Island, where she worked as a management consultant for the North Shore Health System. It was a brisk March morning, and she needed to find somewhere to pull over fast.

As she got off the F.D.R. onto the ramp to the Triborough Bridge, her head was swimming and her stomach was roiling. She was in what scientists call the "prodromal phase of emesis." Salivation increases, sometimes torrentially. The pupils dilate. The heart begins to race. The blood vessels in the skin constrict, increasing pallor—NASA scientists have even used skin sensors to detect space sickness in astronauts, who are sometimes reluctant to admit experiencing nausea. People break out in a cold sweat. Fatigue and often drowsiness occur in minutes. Attention, reflexes, and concentration wane.

While all this is going on, the stomach develops abnormal electrical activity, which prevents it from emptying and causes it to relax. The esophagus contracts, pulling the upper portion of the stomach from the abdomen, through the diaphragm, and into the chest, forming a kind of funnel from stomach to esophagus. Then, in a single movement, known as the "retrograde giant contraction," the upper small intestine evacuates its contents backward into the stomach in preparation for vomiting. In the lower small intestine, smaller rhythmic contractions push the contents into the colon.

As Fitzpatrick came off the exit ramp, the lanes opened out like a fan, and all the drivers around her jockeyed for position. She looked for a place to pull over on the right side of the road, but there wasn't any. She started to cut across the lanes to the left, aiming for a no-man's-land between the traffic going into the toll booths and the traffic coming out from the other direction. She began to retch, and she fished out an empty plastic grocery bag. Then she vomited. Some of the vomit hit the dress and jacket she wore. Some got into the bag she held with one hand. She kept her eyes open and kept the car steady, though, and made it out of the traffic. Then she braked to a halt, bent forward against her shoulder belt, and brought up whatever she had left.

The vomiting act itself has two phases. The retching phase involves a few rounds of coordinated contractions of the abdominal muscles, the diaphragm, and the muscles of respiratory inspiration. So far, nothing has come out. In the expulsive phase, the diaphragm and the abdomen undergo a massive, prolonged contraction, generating intense pressure in the stomach; when the esophagus relaxes, it's as if someone had taken the plug off a fire hydrant.

Vomiting usually makes people feel better, at least for a little while, but Fitzpatrick didn't feel any better. She sat there with the cars rushing by, waiting for the sick feeling to pass, but it didn't. Eventually, still queasy, she drove over the bridge, turned the car around, went home, and climbed into bed. Over the next few days, she began to lose her appetite, and strong odors became intolerable. Easter came that weekend, and she and her husband, Bob, drove down to Alexandria, Virginia, to see her family. She was barely able to tolerate the ride, and had to spend it lying flat on the backseat. It would be months before she could make it back to New York.

At her parents' home, her symptoms rapidly escalated. That weekend, she was unable to hold down any food or liquid at all. She became thoroughly dehydrated. The Monday after Easter, she spent a few hours at the hospital and got replenished with intravenous fluid. She saw her mother's obstetrician, who reassured her that nausea and vomiting were normal during pregnancy, and gave her some common, practical advice: stay away from strong odors and cold liquids, and try to get down small amounts of food whenever possible — perhaps dry crackers and other carbohydrates. Since Fitzpatrick's symptoms were normal, the doctor didn't want to consider prescribing drugs. Pregnancy sickness, she pointed out, usually goes away by the fourteenth, at most the sixteenth, week of pregnancy.

Fitzpatrick was determined, but she found that she couldn't tolerate anything except a bite of cracker or toast. By the end of the week, she needed more hydration, and the doctor arranged for a visiting nurse to come to her parents' house and administer IV fluids. Fitzpatrick continually felt that she was on the verge of throwing up. She had been someone who could eat almost anything; now the smell of the blandest foods made her gag. She had always loved stomach-churning amusement park rides; now riding in a car or just standing up or tilting her head brought on severe motion sickness. She couldn't make it down the stairs. Even in bed, watching TV or focusing on a magazine made her head reel. Over the next couple of weeks, she would vomit five or six times a day. She lost twelve pounds instead of gaining weight, as a woman bearing twins should have. The worst of it was the sense that she was losing control of her life. The management executive in her couldn't stand it. Here she was, back in the house she had grown up in. Her mother had to take a leave from teaching high school to care for her. She felt as if she were a helpless child.

What is nausea, this strange and awful beast? The subject gets little attention in medical school, and yet, after pain, nausea is the most frequent complaint for which people consult physicians. It is a typical side effect of drugs. Among surgery patients, vomiting after anesthesia is so common that an "emesis basin" is kept at the side of every bed in the recovery room. A majority of chemotherapy patients suffer nausea, and they consistently rank it as the worst part of the treatment. From 60 to 85 percent of pregnant women experience morning sickness or "pregnancy sickness," and a third of those who are employed miss work as a result of it. In about five in a thousand pregnant women, the condition is so severe as to cause substantial weight loss—a condition termed "hyperemesis of pregnancy." And, of course, motion sickness afflicts virtually all of us at some point in our lives. Seasickness has been a major military concern dating back to ancient Greece. (The word *nausea* comes from the Greek word for ship.) Cybersickness continues to hobble the development of virtual reality devices. And space sickness is a frequent, though rarely mentioned, problem for astronauts.

The most striking thing about nausea is that it is so intensely aversive (Cicero claimed he "would rather be killed than again suffer the tortures of seasickness"), and not just in the moment. Long after the pain of childbirth fades from memory, mothers will vividly recall their experience of nausea; it is even a reason that some women don't want to bear more children. Nausea is remarkable in this way. Break a leg on a ski slope and—as bad as traumatic pain can be—once you can, you'll ski again. After one unfortunate experience with a bottle of gin or an oyster, by contrast, people won't go near the culprit for years. In Anthony Burgess's *A Clockwork Orange*, the authorities programmed Alex away from brutality by coupling his violent urges with feelings of nausea, not of pain. At one time, some German towns made similar efforts. An 1843 manuscript relates that delinquent juveniles used to be put inside a box outside town hall, whereupon a policeman spun the box around at high speed until the youths had provided the gathered crowd with a "disgusting spectacle."

The sheer loathsomeness of nausea and vomiting does seem to serve a biological purpose. The benefit of vomiting after eating something poisonous or tainted is obvious: the toxin is expelled. And the dreadfulness of the accompanying nausea deters you from ever wanting to eat anything like it again. This explains why pills, chemotherapy, and general anesthetics so often cause nausea and vomiting: they are poisons—albeit controlled ones—and the body is designed to reject them.

Why other things cause nausea and vomiting is more difficult to explain, but scientists are beginning to see some sense in nature's design. You'd think that pregnancy sickness, for example, would be evolutionarily disadvantageous, since a growing embryo needs nutrition. In a famous 1992 paper, however, the evolutionary biologist Margie Profet made a compelling case that pregnancy sickness is actually protective. She pointed out that natural foods that are safe for adults commonly turn out to be unsafe for embryos. All plants produce toxins, and in order to be able to eat them we have evolved elaborate detoxification systems. But these systems don't eliminate harmful chemicals completely, and embryos can be sensitive to even tiny amounts. (For example, toxins in potatoes have been found to cause neural malformations in animal fetuses, even at levels that are nontoxic to their mothers; indeed, Ireland's heavy potato consumption may account for its having the world's highest rate of neural defects, such as spina bifida.)

Pregnancy sickness, Profet suggested, may have evolved to reduce an embryo's exposure to natural toxins. She pointed out that women with pregnancy sickness strongly prefer bland foods that do not spoil easily (like breads and cereals) and are particularly averse to foods associated with high levels of natural toxins, such as bitter or pungent foods and animal products that are not extremely fresh. The theory also explains why sickness occurs mainly during the first trimester. That is when the embryo develops organs and is most sensitive to toxins; at the same time, it is small and its calorie needs are easily supplied by the mother's fat stores. Overall, women with moderate to severe morning sickness have a lower rate of miscarriages than women with mild nausea or none at all.

The purpose of motion sickness is harder to account for. In 1882, the Harvard psychologist William James observed that certain deaf people were immune to seasickness, and since then a great deal of attention has been focused on the role of the vestibular system—the inner ear components that enable us to track our position in space. Scientists came to believe that vigorous motion overstimulates this system, producing signals in the brain that trigger nausea and vomiting. But as Charles Oman, an M.I.T. aerospace physiologist, points out, this theory could not explain many characteristics of motion sickness: why activities like running, jumping, or dancing almost never produce sickness, whereas motion that isn't under your control—for example, being flung around the Gravitron at the county fair—does; why drivers of cars or pilots of aircraft are much less susceptible than passengers; and why sickness tends to diminish with experience. Motion sickness can occur without any motion at all— as with cybersickness or, a related phenomenon, "cinerama sickness," which comes from watching very wide-screen movies. Oman found that among the most provocative stimuli for space sickness in astronauts is simply seeing another astronaut float by upside down, which can produce a sudden, nauseating perception that you are the one who is upside down.

Researchers have now established that motion sickness occurs when there is a conflict between the motion we experience and the motion we expect to experience. Merely to balance our heads on our shoulders, our bodies on our hips and feet, we require an incredibly fine-tuned "body sense"—a system that learns to anticipate motion based on input from vision, muscles, and, especially, the inner ear. Nausea arises when the brain receives unanticipated sensory inputs— for someone new to boats, say, feeling the ground beneath him pitch up and down, or, for someone in a virtual-reality helmet, seeing oneself move through the world while one's body knows it is standing still. (Taking the wheel of a vehicle helps, because one can have more control and feel for how one is moving.) To put it simply, motion sickness is really sickness from unfamiliar motion.

But why does unfamiliar motion make us feel so miserable? A leading explanation returns to the notion of nausea and vomiting as something that protects against toxins. During the Pleistocene epoch, when our species evolved, people had no occasion to experience sustained passive motion, as they do today, on a boat or in a car. Much the same sensation can occur with the ingestion of many hallucinatory toxins, however—as anyone who has drunk too much alcohol can attest. So the nausea and vomiting that comes with motion sickness may be a modern by-product of our standard system for expelling poisons and nurturing avoidance of them. This theory is not nearly as well examined as the explanation for pregnancy sickness, however. And we still don't have a convincing explanation of why anxiety or the sight of blood or of vomit itself should make people sick.

However adaptive nausea and vomiting might be, in cases of hyperemesis like Amy Fitzpatrick's these reflexes seem to spin out of control. Indeed, prior to the Second World War and the development of modern techniques for replacing fluids, hyperemesis was routinely fatal unless the pregnancy was aborted. Even today, although death is rare, serious injury from the severe vomiting can occur—including rupture of the esophagus, lung collapse, and tearing of the spleen. No one would suggest that Fitzpatrick's condition was in the least beneficial. Something had to be done to help her.

Once Fitzpatrick had lost twelve pounds, her doctor prescribed drugs in an effort to control the nausea and vomiting and allow her to eat and drink again. First, the doctor tried Reglan, a drug often used to treat nausea from general anesthesia. Fitzpatrick wore a device that pumped the drug into her leg around the clock. It didn't seem to help, though; instead, it produced frightening neurological side effects—tremors, lockjaw, body rigidity, and difficulty breathing. The doctor tried a second drug, Compazine, which didn't do much of anything, and then still another, Phenergan suppositories, which made her drowsy but didn't slow the vomiting.

All of those drugs work by blocking dopamine receptors in the brain. There is, however, a more recent class of antiemetics on the market today, serotonin-receptor blockers, and these have been hailed as a breakthrough in the treatment of nausea and vomiting. They aren't cheap—Zofran, the biggest seller, costs a hundred and twenty-five dollars a day or more—but studies show that they substantially reduce vomiting in chemotherapy patients and also in some surgery patients. Nor have any problems with birth defects been detected. So Fitzpatrick was given Zofran by vein for several weeks, but, once again, to no avail.

Her doctor also arranged for blood tests, ultrasounds, and consultations with numerous specialists. Nausea can signify an obstruction of the gastrointestinal tract, or a severe infection, or poisoning. But no alternative cause could be found.

"I know the doctors are trying their best," Fitzpatrick would say, and she tried her best, too. She just had to hang in there, she told herself, and, ever the M.B.A., she was organized about it. She arranged for a supply of plastic kidney-shaped emesis basins to be stationed at strategic points around the house, and for a suction apparatus with a plastic nozzle to be kept at her bedside for vacuuming all the sickly saliva from her mouth. For the most part, though, when she wasn't bent over vomiting, she just lay in bed with her eyes closed.

Meanwhile, a small committee of family and friends systematically gathered information on treatment options, both conventional and otherwise. At various points, Fitzpatrick tried herbal therapy, Chinese massage, and water with lemon in it. She tried ginger after she learned about a study showing that it might be effective for her condition. She tried Sea-Bands, which are acupressure wristbands that apply constant pressure at the "Neiguan point"—a spot on the inside of each forearm situated three finger-widths down from the wrist crease, between the tendons. (Though acupressure has been touted for nausea resulting from pregnancy, chemotherapy, and motion, studies have not revealed any consistent effect.) None of it reduced Fitzpatrick's nausea, although she did enjoy the massages.

Even more disturbing, the symptoms weren't getting better with time, as her doctors had expected. By the fourth month of pregnancy, she was as nauseated as she had ever been—an exceedingly unusual occurrence. She looked frighteningly ill. Her weight was down sixteen pounds. Her doctor admitted her to the George Washington University Hospital and had her seen by the high-risk obstetrics service. She was put on intravenous nutrition and she finally started gaining weight. During the next few months, however, she spent more time in the hospital than out.

To her doctors, she was now a spectral, ever-present reminder of failure—the kind of patient whose very existence is a reproach to them and their expertise. Doctors have several ways of dealing with these patients, and in the course of events she must have seen all of them. Some doctors kept telling her that in another week or two she'd turn the corner. One doctor asked if she wanted to go back to New York, and she got the distinct impression that he just wanted to get rid of her. Another seemed to believe that she wasn't trying hard enough to eat, as if the nausea were under her control. Their frustration was palpable. Later, they suggested that she see a psychiatrist.

This was not an unreasonable suggestion. Anxiety and stress can influence nausea, and she was willing to try anything that might help. But Fitzpatrick says that the psychiatrist who saw her kept focusing on whether she was angry at the babies and unable to accept her roles as wife and mother. A surprising number of doctors still believe in the discredited Freudian theory that hyperemesis is due to an unconscious rejection of pregnancy.

The situation had moved beyond the doctors' control and, worse, their understanding. Naturally, Fitzpatrick sought to gain a measure of control herself. At one point, she and her family pushed her team to try a treatment they had come across in an article about Maria Shriver's experience with hyperemesis. The treatment involved a continuous infusion of droperidol, a tranquilizer that is often used to reduce nausea and vomiting in surgery patients. The doctors agreed to try it. During the infusion, however, Fitzpatrick's condition actually worsened. She started throwing up every ten minutes, developed small tears in her esophagus, and began bringing up blood by the cupful.

Her suffering was bottomless. It is not uncommon in hyperemesis cases for women to abort the pregnancy because of the unrelieved misery. A woman across the hall from her did abort because of hyperemesis, and the doctors proposed the same option for Fitzpatrick. She did not consider it, partly because she was an observant Catholic and partly because each day the nurse came by with a small ultrasound device that allowed her to hear the two tiny hearts fluttering inside her womb. Somehow, that was enough to keep her going.

There is no universal antiemetic. Skin patches containing the drug scopolamine reduce motion sickness and postoperative vomiting but seem to do little for pregnant women or chemotherapy patients. The dopamine-receptor antagonist Phenergan works well for many pregnant women and motion-sickness sufferers but not for chemotherapy patients. Even a cutting-edge drug like Zofran, which is often seen as a kind of penicillin for nausea, frequently doesn't help. While Zofran can be highly effective against vomiting from chemotherapy and anesthesia, studies show that it doesn't help with motion sickness or hyperemesis of pregnancy. (Smoking marijuana, by the way, appears to be effective for chemotherapy patients, if only weakly, but in pregnancy it is as toxic for the fetus as tobacco is.)

This makes sense when you recall that nausea is a condition that can be triggered by stimuli as different as an unfamiliar motion, a bad smell, a toxic drug, and the hormonal fluctuations of pregnancy. As scientists explain it, the brain has a vomiting program (or "module") that receives and responds to all kinds of inputs: from chemoreceptors in the nose, the gut, and the brain; from receptors that detect overfilling of the stomach or tickling of the uvula; from motion sensors in the inner ear; and from higher brain centers governing memory, mood, and cognition. Each of our current drugs presumably interferes with some pathways more than with others. Hence the different effects in different conditions.

What's more, although we often think of nausea and vomiting as part of the same phenomenon, they are quite separate, probably involving separate programs in the brain, and a drug that affects one may not affect the other. Vomiting does not always involve nausea. I can remember a kid in sixth grade who could vomit at will—no finger down the throat or anything—even though he didn't feel the least bit sick. And people with the rare condition known as rumination syndrome have an unexplained tendency to vomit food up from their stomach into their mouth shortly after every meal—this without any associated nausea. (They either swallow the food again or spit it out, "depending on social circumstances," as one scientific article put it.) Conversely, even severe nausea does not necessarily produce vomiting. And drugs that stop vomiting do not necessarily stop nausea—a point that many doctors and nurses often fail to recognize. For example, people working in medicine have been highly impressed by Zofran, but patients may be less so. A study led by Gary Morrow, a nausea researcher at the University of Rochester Medical School, found that widespread use of Zofran and its cousins had reduced vomiting in chemotherapy patients but had produced no improvement in the severity of their nausea. In fact, patients today report having a longer duration of nausea than patients had during the pre-Zofran years.

Researchers studying chemotherapy patients—a sort of captive population for scientists investigating how nausea and vomiting occur—have discovered something even more surprising. These patients actually experience three separate types of nausea and vomiting. An "acute" type occurs within minutes to hours of receiving a dose of a toxic chemotherapy drug and then gradually resolves— exactly the effect we'd predict from a poison. But then in many patients the nausea and vomiting come back after a day or two, an effect called "delayed emesis." And about a quarter of chemotherapy patients even begin to have "anticipatory nausea and vomiting," symptoms that occur before the drugs are injected. Morrow has documented some striking characteristics of these types of nausea. The more intense the initial acute nausea, the worse the anticipatory nausea becomes. And the more cycles of chemotherapy that patients receive, the more general the cues for anticipatory nausea become: vomiting may occur first when a patient sees the nurse who administers the drugs, then when he sees any nurse or takes in the smell of the clinic, then when he pulls into the clinic parking lot for his chemotherapy appointment. Morrow had one patient who vomited whenever she saw the highway exit sign for the hospital.

These reactions are, of course, familiar results of psychological conditioning—the "Clockwork Orange" effect in action. Such conditioning probably plays an important role in prolonging nausea in other circumstances, including pregnancy. Once delayed or anticipatory vomiting develops, though, current drugs don't help. Studies by Morrow and others have found that only behavioral treatments, like hypnosis or deep relaxation techniques, significantly reduce conditioned vomiting, and then only for some patients.

Ultimately, our medical arsenal against nausea and vomiting is still fairly primitive. Given how common these problems are and how much people are willing to pay to make them go away, pharmaceutical companies are investing millions of dollars in efforts to find more effective drugs. Merck, for example, has developed a promising contender, currently known as MK-869. This is one of a new class of agents called "substance P antagonists." These drugs attracted a good deal of attention when Merck announced that they seemed to be clinically effective against depression. Less noted, however, were findings published in the *New England Journal of Medicine* that MK-869 was remarkably effective against nausea and vomiting in chemotherapy patients.

The findings were unusual for two reasons. First, the drug substantially reduced both acute and delayed vomiting. Second, MK-869 didn't just work against vomiting but reduced nausea as well. The proportion of patients reporting anything more than minimal nausea in the five days following chemotherapy dropped from 75 percent to 51 percent with the drug.

All our medications have their limitations, however, and as promising as such new drugs may seem they will fail many patients. Not even MK-869 could stop nausea for half of the chemotherapy patients. (In addition, its safety and effectiveness in pregnant women are likely to remain unknown for some time. Because of both medical and legal hazards, drug companies generally avoid testing drugs on pregnant women.) So there's no morphine for nausea on the horizon. Uncontrolled nausea remains a persistent problem. Still, a brand-new clinical specialty called "palliative medicine" is pursuing a radical project: the scientific study of suffering. And what's striking is that they're finding solutions where others have not.

Palliative specialists are experts in the care of dying patients—specifically in improving the quality of their lives rather than prolonging their lives. One might think we wouldn't need a specialty for this, but there's evidence that these specialists really are better at it. Dying patients often have pain. Many have nausea. Some have such poor lung function that, although they take in enough oxygen to survive, they live with a constant, terrifying breathlessness—a feeling that they are drowning and just cannot get enough air. These are patients with untreatable disease, and yet palliative specialists have been remarkably successful at helping them. The key is simply that they take suffering seriously, as a problem in itself. In medicine, we're used to seeing such symptoms only as clues in a puzzle about where the disease is and what we can do about it. And, as a rule, fixing what's physically wrong—taking out the infected appendix, setting the broken bone, treating the pneumonia—is precisely the way to relieve suffering. (I wouldn't be a surgeon if I thought otherwise.) But not always—and nowhere is this more apparent than with nausea. Most of the time, nausea is not a sign of pathology but a normal response to something like travel or pregnancy—or even to a beneficial treatment like chemotherapy or antibiotics or general anesthesia. The patient, we say, is "fine," but the suffering is no less.

Consider the significance of vital signs. When a patient is in the hospital, every four hours or so a nurse records the vital signs on a bedside chart to provide caregivers with a measure of how the patient is doing over time. This is done the same way the world over. By convention, the four vital signs are temperature, blood pressure, pulse, and respiratory rate. And these do tell us a lot about whether someone is getting physically better or worse. But they don't tell us anything about suffering, about something more than just how the body is doing. Palliative specialists are trying to change this. They want to make pain—the level of discomfort a patient reports—the fifth vital sign. The fuss they've raised is forcing physicians to recognize how often we undertreat pain. And they are developing better treatment strategies generally. For example, it is now evident that, once symptoms of severe nausea (or, for that matter, pain) develop and progress, they become increasingly resistant to therapies of any kind. The best approach, palliative specialists have learned, is to start treatment when the symptoms are mild—or, in some circumstances, even before they appear—and that proves true whether you're a passenger about to board a ship or a cancer patient about to start chemotherapy. (The American Society of Clinical Oncology has announced guidelines endorsing this preventive approach for chemotherapy patients.) Back when doctors didn't hesitate to prescribe antiemetics for ordinary pregnancy sickness—at least a third of pregnant women were on such drugs in the 1960s and 1970s—hyperemesis was much less common. But doctors changed this practice after lawsuits forced the popular remedy Bendectin off the market alleging it caused birth defects (despite numerous studies showing no evidence of harm). It became standard to avoid prescribing drugs until, as in Fitzpatrick's case, vomiting had already caused significant dehydration or starvation. Hospital admissions for hyperemesis of pregnancy subsequently doubled.

Perhaps the most striking observation palliative specialists make, however, is that there is a distinction between symptom and suffering. As the physician Eric J. Cassell points out in his book *The Nature of Suffering and the Goals of Medicine*, for some patients simply receiving a measure of understanding—of knowing what the source of the misery is, seeing its meaning in a different way, or just coming to accept that we cannot always tame nature—can be enough to control their suffering. A doctor can still help, even when medications have failed.

Amy Fitzpatrick said that the doctors she liked best were the few who admitted they didn't know how to explain her nausea or what to do about it. They would say that they had never seen anything like her case, and she could tell that they commiserated with her. She did acknowledge having some contradictory feelings about such admissions. At times, they made her wonder if she had the right doctors, if, somehow, they were missing something. But, for all the treatments she and the doctors tried, the nausea would not let up. It really did seem beyond anyone's comprehension.

The first months were a terrible, frightening struggle. Gradually, though, she felt a transformation, a toughening of her spirit, and she sometimes even had a thought that things were not so bad after all. She prayed every day and believed that the two children growing inside her were a gift from God, and, with time, she came to see her trials as simply the price she had to pay for this remarkable joy. She gave up looking for silver bullets. After the twenty-sixth week of pregnancy, she asked for no more experimental therapies. The nausea and the vomiting persisted, but she would not be defeated by them.

Eventually, there was a glimmer of relief. By the thirtieth week, she found that she could eat an odd selection of four things in sliver-size portions: steak, asparagus, tuna, and mint ice cream. And she was able to hold down a protein drink. The nausea remained, but it had eased just a bit. In the thirty-third week, seven weeks early, Fitzpatrick went into active labor. Her husband flew down on the shuttle from LaGuardia in time for the delivery. The doctors warned her that the twins would be small, around three pounds, but on September 12, at 10:52 P.M., Linda was born, weighing four pounds twelve ounces, and at 10:57 P.M. Jack was born, at five pounds even—both in excellent health.

Shortly after delivery, Fitzpatrick threw up once more. "But that was the last time," she recalled. The next morning, she drank a big glass of orange juice. And that night she ate a giant hamburger with blue cheese and fries. "It was delicious," she said.

Crimson Tide

In January of 1997, Christine Drury became the overnight anchor-woman for *Channel 13 News*, the local NBC affiliate in Indianapolis. In the realm of television news and talk shows, this is how you get your start. (David Letterman began his career by doing weekend weather at the same station.) Drury worked the 9 P.M. to 5 A.M. shift, developing stories and, after midnight, reading a thirty-second and a two-and-a-half-minute bulletin. If she was lucky and there was break-ing news in the middle of the night, she could get more airtime, cov-ering the news live, either from the newsroom or in the field. If she was very lucky—like the time a Conrail train derailed in Green-castle—she'd get to stay on for the morning show.

Drury was twenty-six years old when she got the job. From the time she was a girl growing up in Kokomo, Indiana, she had wanted to be on television, and especially to be an anchorwoman. She envied the confidence and poise of the women she saw behind the desk. One day during high school, on a shopping trip to an Indianapolis mall, she spotted Kim Hood, who was then Channel 13's prime-time anchor. "I wanted to be her," Drury says, and the encounter somehow made the goal seem attainable. In college, at Purdue University, she majored in telecommunications, and one summer she did an internship at Channel 13. A year and a half after graduating, she landed a bottom-rung job there as a production assistant. She ran the TelePrompTer, positioned cameras, and generally did whatever she was told. During the next two years, she worked her way up to writing news and then, finally, to the overnight anchor job. Her bosses saw her as an ideal prospect. She wrote fine news scripts, they told her, had a TV-ready voice, and, not incidentally, had "the look"—which is to say that she was pretty in a wholesome, all-American, Meg Ryan way. She had perfect white teeth, blue eyes, blond hair, and an easy smile.

During her broadcasts, however, she found that she could not stop blushing. The most inconsequential event was enough to set it off. She'd be on the set, reading the news, and then she'd stumble over a word or realize that she was talking too fast. Almost instantly, she'd redden. A sensation of electric heat would start in her chest and then surge upward into her neck, her ears, her scalp. In physiological terms, it was a mere redirection of blood flow. The face and neck have an unusual number of veins near the surface, and they can carry more blood than those of similar size elsewhere. Stimulated by certain neurological signals, they will dilate while other peripheral vessels contract: the hands will turn white and clammy even as the face flushes. For Drury, more troubling than the physical reaction was the distress that accompanied it: her mind would go blank; she'd hear herself stammer. She'd have an overwhelming urge to cover her face with her hands, to turn away from the camera, to hide.

For as long as Drury could remember, she had been a blusher, and, with her pale Irish skin, her blushes stood out. She was the sort of child who almost automatically reddened with embarrassment when called on in class or while searching for a seat in the school lunchroom. As an adult, she could be made to blush by a grocery-store cashier's holding up the line to get a price on her cornflakes, or by getting honked at while driving. It may seem odd that such a person would place herself in front of a camera. But Drury had always fought past her tendency toward embarrassment. In high school, she had been a cheerleader, played on the tennis team, and been selected for the prom-queen court. At Purdue, she had played intramural tennis, rowed crew with friends, and graduated Phi Beta Kappa. She'd worked as a waitress and as an assistant manager at a Wal-Mart, even leading the staff every morning in the Wal-Mart cheer. Her gregariousness and social grace had always assured her a large circle of friends.

On the air, though, she was not getting past the blushing. When you look at tapes of her early broadcasts—reporting on an increase in speeding-ticket fines, a hotel food poisoning, a twelve-year-old with an IQ of 325 who graduated from college—the redness is clearly visible. Later, she began wearing turtlenecks and applying to her face a thick layer of Merle Norman Cover Up Green concealer. Over this she would apply MAC Studiofix foundation. Her face ended up a bit dark, but the redness became virtually unnoticeable.

Still, a viewer could tell that something wasn't right. Now when she blushed—and eventually she would blush nearly every other broadcast—you could see her stiffen, her eyes fixate, her movements become mechanical. Her voice sped up and rose in pitch. "She was a real deer in the headlights," one producer at the station said.

Drury gave up caffeine. She tried breath-control techniques. She bought self-help books for television performers and pretended the camera was her dog, her friend, her mom. For a while, she tried holding her head a certain way, very still, while on camera. Nothing worked.

Given the hours and the extremely limited exposure, being an overnight anchor is a job without great appeal. People generally do it for about a year, perfect their skills, and move on to a better position. But Drury was going nowhere. "She was definitely not ready to be on during daylight hours," the producer said. In October of 1998, almost two years into her job, she wrote in her journal, "My feelings of slipping continue. I spent the entire day crying. I'm on my way to work and I feel like I may never use enough Kleenex. I can't figure out why God would bless me with a job I can't do. I have to figure out how to do it. I'll try everything before I give up."

What is this peculiar phenomenon called blushing? A skin reaction? An emotion? A kind of vascular expression? Scientists have never been sure how to describe it. The blush is at once physiology and psychology. On the one hand, blushing is involuntary, uncontrollable, and external, like a rash. On the other hand, it requires thought and feeling at the highest order of cerebral function. "Man is the only animal that blushes," Mark Twain wrote. "Or needs to."

Observers have often assumed that blushing is simply the outward manifestation of shame. Freudians, for example, viewed blushing this way, arguing that it is a displaced erection, resulting from repressed sexual desire. But, as Darwin noted and puzzled over in an 1872 essay, it is not shame but the prospect of exposure, of humiliation, that makes us blush. "A man may feel thoroughly ashamed at having told a small falsehood, without blushing," he wrote, "but if he even suspects that he is detected he will instantly blush, especially if detected by one whom he reveres."

But if it is humiliation that we are concerned about, why do we blush when we're praised? Or when people sing "Happy Birthday" to us? Or when people just look at us? Michael Lewis, a professor of psychiatry at the University of Medicine and Dentistry of New Jersey, routinely demonstrates the effect in classes. He announces that he will randomly point at a student, that the pointing is meaningless and reflects no judgment whatever about the person. Then he closes his eyes and points. Everyone looks to see who it is. And, invariably, that person is overcome by embarrassment. In an odd experiment conducted a couple of years ago, two social psychologists, Janice Templeton and Mark Leary, wired subjects with facial-temperature sensors and put them on one side of a one-way mirror. The mirror was then removed to reveal an entire audience staring at them from the other side. Half the time the audience members were wearing dark glasses, and half the time they were not. Strangely, subjects blushed only when they could see the audience's eyes.

What is perhaps most disturbing about blushing is that it produces secondary effects of its own. It is itself embarrassing, and can cause intense self-consciousness, confusion, and loss of focus. (Darwin, struggling to explain why this might be, conjectured that the greater blood flow to the face drained blood from the brain.)

Why we have such a reflex is perplexing. One theory is that the blush exists to show embarrassment, just as the smile exists to show happiness. This would explain why the reaction appears only in the visible regions of the body (the face, the neck, and the upper chest). But then why do dark-skinned people blush? Surveys find that nearly everyone blushes, regardless of skin color, despite the fact that in many people it is nearly invisible. And you don't need to turn red in order for people to recognize that you're embarrassed. Studies show that people detect embarrassment *before* you blush. Apparently, blushing takes between fifteen and twenty seconds to reach its peak, yet most people need less than five seconds to recognize that someone is embarrassed—they pick it up from the almost immediate shift in gaze, usually down and to the left, or from the sheepish, self-conscious grin that follows a half second to a second later. So there's reason to doubt that the purpose of blushing is entirely expressive.

There is, however, an alternative view held by a growing number of scientists. The effect of intensifying embarrassment may not be incidental; perhaps that is what blushing is for. The notion isn't as absurd as it sounds. People may hate being embarrassed and strive not to show it when they are, but embarrassment serves an important good. For, unlike sadness or anger or even love, it is fundamentally a moral emotion. Arising from sensitivity to what others think, embarrassment provides painful notice that one has crossed certain bounds while at the same time providing others with a kind of apology. It keeps us in good standing in the world. And if blushing serves to heighten such sensitivity, this may be to one's ultimate advantage.

The puzzle, though, is how to shut it off. Embarrassment causes blushing, and blushing causes embarrassment—so what makes the cycle stop? No one knows, but in some people the mechanism clearly goes awry. A surprisingly large number of people experience frequent, severe, uncontrollable blushing. They describe it as "intense," "random," and "mortifying." One man I talked to would blush even when he was at home by himself just watching somebody get embarrassed on TV, and he lost his job as a management consultant because his bosses thought he didn't seem "comfortable" with clients. Another man, a neuroscientist, left a career in clinical medicine for a cloistered life in research almost entirely because of his tendency to blush. And even then he could not get away from it. His work on hereditary brain disease became so successful that he found himself fending off regular invitations to give talks and to appear on TV. He once hid in an office bathroom to avoid a CNN crew. On another occasion, he was invited to present his work to fifty of the world's top scientists, including five Nobel Prize winners. Usually, he could get through a talk by turning off the lights and showing slides. But this time a member of the audience stopped him with a question first, and the neuroscientist went crimson. He stood mumbling for a moment, then retreated behind the podium and surreptitiously activated his pager. He looked down at it and announced that an emergency had come up. He was very sorry, he said, but he had to go. He spent the rest of the day at home. This is someone who makes his living studying disorders of the brain and the nerves. Yet he could not make sense of his own condition.

There is no official name for this syndrome, though it is often called "severe" or "pathological" blushing, and no one knows how many people have it. One very crude estimate suggests that from 1 to 7 percent of the general population is afflicted. Unlike most people, whose blushing diminishes after their teenage years, chronic blushers report an increase as they age. At first, it was thought that the problem was the intensity of their blushing. But that proved not to be the case. In one study, for example, scientists used sensors to monitor the facial color and temperature of subjects, then made them stand before an audience and do things like sing "The Star-Spangled Banner" or dance to a song. Chronic blushers became no redder than others, but they proved significantly more prone to blush. Christine Drury described the resulting vicious cycle to me: one fears blushing, blushes, and then blushes at being so embarrassed about blushing. Which came first—the blushing or the embarrassment—she did not know. She just wanted it to stop.

In the fall of 1998, Drury went to see an internist. "You'll grow out of it," he told her. When she pressed, however, he agreed to let her try medication. It couldn't have been obvious what to prescribe. Medical textbooks say nothing about pathological blushing. Some doctors prescribe anxiolytics, like Valium, on the assumption that the real problem is anxiety. Some prescribe beta-blockers, which blunt the body's stress response. Some prescribe Prozac or other anti-depressants. The one therapy that has been shown to have modest success is not a drug but a behavioral technique known as paradoxical intention—having patients actively try to blush instead of trying not to. Drury used beta-blockers first, then antidepressants, and finally psychotherapy. There was no improvement.

By December of 1998, her blushing had become intolerable, her on-air performance humiliating, and her career almost unsalvageable. She wrote in her diary that she was ready to resign. Then one day she searched the Internet for information about facial blushing, and read about a hospital in Sweden where doctors were performing a surgical procedure that could stop it. The operation involved severing certain nerves in the chest where they exit the spinal cord to travel up to the head. "I'm reading this page about people who have the exact same problem I had, and I couldn't believe it," she told me. "Tears were streaming down my face." The next day, she told her father that she had decided to have the surgery. Mr. Drury seldom questioned his daughter's choices, but this sounded to him like a bad idea. "It shocked me, really," he recalls. "And when she told her mother it shocked her even worse. There was basically no way her daughter was going to Sweden and having this operation."

Drury agreed to take some time to learn more about the surgery. She read the few articles she could find in medical journals. She spoke to the surgeons and to former patients. After a couple of weeks, she grew only more convinced. She told her parents that she was going to Sweden, and when it became clear that she would not be deterred her father decided to go with her.

The surgery is known as endoscopic thoracic sympathectomy, or ETS. It involves severing fibers of a person's sympathetic nervous system, part of the involuntary, or "autonomic," nervous system, which controls breathing, heart rate, digestion, sweating, and, among the many other basic functions of life, blushing. Toward the back of your chest, running along either side of the spine like two smooth white strings, are the sympathetic trunks, the access roads that sympathetic nerves travel along before exiting to individual organs. At the beginning of the twentieth century, surgeons tried removing branches of these trunks—a thoracic sympathectomy—for all sorts of conditions: epilepsy, glaucoma, certain cases of blindness. Mostly, the experiments did more harm than good. But surgeons did find two unusual instances in which a sympathectomy helped: it stopped intractable chest pain in patients with advanced, inoperable heart disease, and it put an end to hand and facial sweating in patients with hyperhidrosis—uncontrollable sweating.

Because the operation traditionally required opening the chest, it was rarely performed. In recent years, however, a few surgeons, particularly in Europe, have been doing the procedure endoscopically, using scopes inserted through small incisions. Among them was a trio in Göteborg, Sweden, who noticed that many of their hyperhidrosis patients not only stopped sweating after surgery but stopped blushing, too. In 1992, the Göteborg group accepted a handful of patients who complained of disabling blushing. When the results were reported in the press, the doctors found themselves deluged with requests. Since 1998, the surgeons have done the operation for more than three thousand patients with severe blushing.

The operation is now performed around the world, but the Göteborg surgeons are among the few to have published their results: 94 percent of their patients reported experiencing a substantial reduction in blushing; in most cases it was eliminated completely. In surveys taken some eight months after the surgery, 2 percent regretted the decision, because of side effects, and 15 percent were dissatisfied. The side effects are not life-threatening, but they are not trivial. The most serious injury, occurring in 1 percent of patients, is Horner's syndrome, in which inadvertent damage to the sympathetic nerves feeding the eye results in a constricted pupil, a drooping eyelid, and a sunken eyeball. Less seriously, patients no longer sweat from the nipples upward, and most experience a substantial increase in lower-body sweating in compensation. (According to a longer-range study that surveyed hand-sweating patients a decade after undergoing ETS, the proportion who were satisfied with the outcome drops to only 67 percent, mainly because of the compensatory sweating.) About a third of patients also notice a curious reaction known as gustatory sweating—sweating prompted by certain tastes or smells. And, because sympathetic branches to the heart are removed, patients experience about a 10 percent reduction in heart rate; some complain of impaired physical performance. For all these reasons, the operation is at best a last resort, something to be tried, according to the surgeons, only after nonsurgical methods have failed. By the time people call Göteborg, they are often desperate. As one patient who had the operation told me, "I would have gone through with it even if they told me there was a fifty percent chance of death."

On January 14, 1999, Christine Drury and her father arrived in Göteborg. The city is a four-hundred-year-old seaport on Sweden's southwest coast, and she remembers the day as cold, snowy, and beautiful. The Carlanderska Medical Center was old and small, with ivy-covered walls and big, arched wooden double doors. Inside, it was dim and silent; Drury was reminded of a dungeon. Only now did she become apprehensive, wondering what she was doing here, nine thousand miles away from home, at a hospital that she knew almost nothing about. Still, she checked in, and a nurse drew her blood for routine lab tests, made sure her medical records were in order, and took her payment, which came to six thousand dollars. Drury put it on a credit card.

The hospital room was reassuringly clean and modern, with white linens and blue blankets. Christer Drott, her surgeon, came to see her early the next morning. He spoke with impeccable British-accented English and was, she said, exceedingly comforting: "He holds your hand and is so compassionate. Those doctors have seen thousands of these cases. I just loved him."

At nine-thirty that morning, an orderly came to get her for the operation. "We had just done a story about a kid who died because the anesthesiologist had fallen asleep," Drury says. "So I made sure to ask the anesthesiologist not to fall asleep and let me die. He kind of laughed and said, 'OK.'"

While Drury was unconscious, Drott, in scrubs and sterile gown, swabbed her chest and axillae (underarms) with antiseptic and laid down sterile drapes so that only her axillae were exposed. After feeling for a space between the ribs in her left axilla, he made a seven-millimeter puncture with the tip of his scalpel, then pushed a large-bore needle through the hole and into her chest. Two liters of carbon dioxide were pumped in through the needle, pushing her left lung downward and out of the way. Then Drott inserted a resecto-scope, a long metal tube fitted with an eyepiece, fiber-optic illumi-nation, and a cauterizing tip. It is actually a urological instrument, thin enough to pass through the urethra (though never thin enough, of course, for urology patients). Looking through the lens, he searched for her left sympathetic trunk, taking care to avoid injuring the main blood vessels from her heart, and found the glabrous, cordlike structure lying along the heads of her ribs, where they join the spine. He cauterized the trunk at two points, over the second and third ribs, destroying all the facial branches except those that lead to the eye. Then, after making sure there was no bleeding, he pulled the instrument out, inserted a catheter to suction out the carbon dioxide and let her lung re-expand, and sutured the quarter-inch incision. Moving to the other side of the table, he performed the same procedure on the right side of her chest. Everything went without a hitch. The operation took just twenty minutes.

What happens when you take away a person's ability to blush? Is it merely a surgical version of Merle Norman Cover Up Green—removing the redness but not the self-consciousness? Or can a few snips of peripheral nerve fibers actually affect the individual herself? I remember once, as a teenager, buying mirrored sunglasses. I lost them within a few weeks, but when I had them on I found myself staring at people brazenly, acting a little tougher. I felt disguised behind those glasses, less exposed, somehow freer. Would the surgery be something like that?

Almost two years after Drury's operation, I had lunch with her at a sports bar in Indianapolis. I had been wondering what her face would look like without the nerves that are meant to control its coloring—would she look ashen, blotchy, unnatural in some way? In fact, her face is clear and slightly pinkish, no different, she said, from before. Yet, since the surgery, she has not blushed. Occasionally, almost randomly, she has experienced a phantom blush: a distinct feeling that she is blushing even though she is not. I asked if her face reddens when she runs, and she said no, although it will if she stands on her head. The other physical changes seemed minor to her. The most noticeable thing, she said, was that neither her face nor her arms sweat now and her stomach, back, and legs sweat much more than they used to, though not enough to bother her. The scars, tiny to begin with, have completely disappeared.

From the first morning after the operation, Drury says, she felt transformed. An attractive male nurse came to take her blood pressure. Ordinarily, she would have blushed the instant he approached. But nothing of the sort happened. She felt, she says, as if a mask had been removed.

That day, after being discharged, she put herself to the test, asking random people on the street for directions, a situation that had invariably caused her to redden. Now, as her father confirmed, she didn't. What's more, the encounters felt easy and ordinary, without a glimmer of her old self-consciousness. At the airport, she recalls, she and her father were waiting in a long check-in line and she couldn't find her passport. "So I just dumped my purse out onto the floor and started looking for it, and it occurred to me that I was doing this — and I wasn't mortified," she says. "I looked up at my dad and just started crying."

Back home, the world seemed new. Attention now felt uncomplicated, unfrightening. Her usual internal monologue when talking to people ("Please don't blush, please don't blush, oh God I'm going to blush") vanished, and she found that she could listen to others better. She could look at them longer, too, without the urge to avert her gaze. (In fact, she had to teach herself not to stare.)

Five days after the surgery, Drury was back at the anchor desk. She put on almost no makeup that night. She wore a navy-blue woolen blazer, the kind of warm clothing she would never have worn before. "My attitude was, This is my debut," she told me. "And it went perfectly."

Later, I viewed some tapes of her broadcasts from the first weeks after the surgery. I saw her report on the killing of a local pastor by a drunk driver, and on the shooting of a nineteen-year-old by a sixteen-year-old. She was more natural than she'd ever been. One broadcast in particular struck me. It was not her regular nighttime bulletin but a public-service segment called "Read, Indiana, Read!" For six minutes of live airtime on a February morning, she was shown reading a story to a crowd of obstreperous eight-year-olds as messages encouraging parents to read to their children scrolled by. Despite the chaos of kids walking by, throwing things, putting their faces up to the camera, she persevered, remaining composed the entire time.

Drury had told no one about the operation, but people at work immediately noticed a difference in her. I spoke to a producer at her station who said, "She just told me she was going on a trip with her dad, but when she came back and I saw her on TV again, I said, 'Christine! That was unbelievable!' She looked amazingly comfortable in front of the camera. You could see the confidence coming through the TV, which was completely different from before." Within months, Drury got a job as a prime-time on-air reporter at another station.

A few snips of fibers to her face and she was changed. It's an odd notion, because we think of our essential self as being distinct from such corporeal details. Who hasn't seen a photo of himself, or heard his voice on tape, and thought, That isn't me! Burn patients who see themselves in a mirror for the first time—to take an extreme example—typically feel alien from their appearance. And yet they do not merely "get used" to it; their new skin changes them. It alters how they relate to people, what they expect of others, how they see themselves in others' eyes. A burn-ward nurse once told me that the secure may become fearful and bitter, the weak jut-jawed "survivors." Similarly, Drury had experienced her trip-wire blushing as something entirely external, not unlike a burn—"the red mask," she called it. Yet it reached so deep inside her that she believed it prevented her from being the person she was meant to be. Once the mask was removed, she seemed new, bold, "completely different from before." But what of the person who all her life had been made embarrassed and self-conscious at the slightest scrutiny? That person, Drury gradually discovered, was still there.

One night, she went out to dinner with a friend and decided to tell him about the operation. He was the first person outside her family she had told, and he was horrified. She'd had an operation to *eliminate her ability to blush?* It seemed warped, he said, and, worse, vain. "You TV people will do anything to improve your career prospects," she recalls him saying.

She went home in tears, angry but also mortified, wondering whether it *was* a freakish and weak thing to have done. In later weeks and months, she became more and more convinced that her surgical solution made her a sort of impostor. "The operation had cleared my path to be the journalist I was trained to be," she says, "but I felt incredibly ashamed over needing to remove my difficulties by such artificial means."

She became increasingly fearful that others would find out about the operation. Once, a coworker, trying to figure out what exactly seemed different about her, asked her if she had lost weight. Smiling weakly, she told him no, and said nothing more. "I remember going to a station picnic the Saturday before the Indy 500, and thinking to myself the whole time, Please, please let me get out of here without anyone saying, 'Hey, what happened to your blushing?'" It was, she found, precisely the same embarrassment as before, only now it stemmed not from blushing but from its absence.

On television, self-consciousness began to distract her again. In June of 1999, she took up her new job, but she was not scheduled to go on the air for two months. During the hiatus, she grew uncertain about going back on TV. One day that summer, she went out with a crew that was covering storm damage in a neighboring town where trees had been uprooted. They let her practice her standup before the camera. She is sure she looked fine, but that wasn't how she felt. "I felt like I didn't belong there, didn't deserve to be there," she says. A few days later, she resigned.

More than a year has passed since then, and Drury has had to spend this time getting her life back on track. Unemployed and ashamed, she withdrew, saw no one, and spent her days watching TV from her couch, in a state of growing depression. Matters changed for her only gradually. She began, against all her instincts, admitting to friends and then former coworkers what had happened. To her surprise and relief, nearly everyone was supportive. In September 1999, she even started an organization, the Red Mask Foundation, to spread information about chronic blushing and to provide a community for its sufferers. Revealing her secret seemed to allow her finally to move on.

That winter, she found a new job—in radio, this time, which made perfect sense. She became the assistant bureau chief for Metro Networks radio in Indianapolis. She could be heard anchoring the news every weekday morning on two radio stations, and then doing the afternoon traffic report for these and several other stations. The next spring, having regained her confidence, she began contacting television stations. The local Fox station agreed to let her be a substitute broadcaster. In early July, she was called in at the last minute to cover traffic on its three-hour morning show.

I got to watch the show on tape. It was one of those breakfast news programs with two chirpy co-anchors—a man and a woman—in overstuffed chairs, cradling giant coffee mugs. Every half hour or so, they'd turn to Drury for a two-minute traffic report. She'd stand before a series of projected city maps, clicking through them and describing the various car accidents and construction roadblocks to look out for. Now and then, the co-anchors would strike up some hey-you're-not-our-usual-traffic-gal banter, which she managed comfortably, laughing and joking. It was exciting, she says, but not easy. She could not help feeling a little self-conscious, wondering what people might think about her coming back after her long absence. But the feelings did not overwhelm her. She is, she says, beginning to feel comfortable in her own skin.

One wants to know whether, in the end, her troubles were physical or psychological. But it is a question as impossible to answer as whether a blush is physical or mental—or, for that matter, whether a person is. Everyone is both, inseparable even by a surgeon's blade. I have asked Drury if she has any regrets about the operation. "Not at all," she says. She even calls the surgery "my cure." At the same time, she adds, "People need to know—surgery isn't the end of it." She has now reached what she describes as a happy medium. She is free from much of the intense self-consciousness that her blushing provoked, but she accepts the fact that she will never be entirely rid of it. The following October, she became a freelance part-time on-air reporter for Channel 6, the ABC television affiliate in Indianapolis. She hopes the job will become full-time.

The Man Who Couldn't Stop Eating

A Roux-en-Y gastric-bypass operation is a radical procedure and the most drastic means available to lose weight. It is also the strangest operation I have ever participated in in surgery. It removes no disease, repairs no defect or injury. It is an operation that is intended to control a person's will—to manipulate a person's innards so that he will not overeat again. And it is soaring in popularity. Some 45,000 obesity patients had gastric-bypass surgery in the United States in 1999, and this number is on its way to doubling by 2003. Vincent Caselli was about to join them.

At 7:30 A.M. on September 13, 1999, an anesthesiologist and two orderlies brought Caselli (whose name has been changed) into the operating room where I and his attending surgeon awaited him. Caselli was fifty-four years old, a heavy-machine operator and road construction contractor (he and his men had paved a rotary in my own neighborhood), the son of Italian immigrants, a husband of thirty-five years, and a father to three girls, all grown now with children of their own. He also weighed four hundred and twenty-eight pounds, though he stood just five feet seven inches tall, and he was miserable. Housebound, his health failing, he no longer had anything resembling a normal life.

For the very obese, general anesthesia alone is a dangerous undertaking; major abdominal surgery can easily become a disaster. Obesity substantially increases the risk of respiratory failure, heart attacks, wound infections, hernias—almost every complication possible, including death. Nevertheless, Dr. Sheldon Randall, the attending surgeon, was relaxed—chatting with the nurses about their weekends, reassuring Caselli that things would go fine—having done more than a thousand of these operations. I, the assisting resident, remained anxious. Watching Caselli struggle to shift himself from the stretcher onto the operating table and then stop halfway to catch his breath, I was afraid that he would fall in between. Once he was on the table, his haunches rolled off the sides, and I double-checked the padding that protected him from the table's sharp edges. He was naked except for his "universal"-size johnny, which covered him like a napkin, and a nurse put a blanket over his lower body for the sake of modesty. When we tried to lay him down, he lost his breath and started to turn blue, and the anesthesiologist had to put him to sleep sitting up. Only with the breathing tube in place and a mechanical ventilator regulating his breathing were we able to lay him flat.

He was a mountain on the table. I am six feet two, but even with the table as low as it goes I had to stand on a step stool to operate; Dr. Randall stood on two stools stacked together. He nodded to me, and I cut down the middle of our patient's belly, through skin and then dense inches of glistening yellow fat. Inside his abdomen, his liver was streaked with fat, too, and his bowel was covered by a thick apron of it, but his stomach looked ordinary—a smooth, grayish-pink bag the size of two fists. We put metal retractors in place to hold the wound open and keep the liver and the slithering loops of bowel out of the way. Working elbow deep, we stapled his stomach down to the size of an ounce. Before the operation, it could accommodate a quart of food and drink; now it would hold no more than a shot glass. We then sewed the opening of this little pouch to a portion of bowel two feet past his duodenum—past the initial portion of the small bowel, where bile and pancreatic juices break food down. This was the bypass part of the operation, and it meant that what food the stomach could accommodate would be less readily absorbed.

The operation took us a little over two hours. Caselli was stable throughout, but his recovery was difficult. Patients are usually ready to go home three days after surgery; it was two days before Caselli even knew where he was. For twenty-four hours, his kidneys stopped working, and fluid built up in his lungs. He became delirious, seeing things on the walls, pulling off his oxygen mask, his chest leads for the monitors, even yanking out the IV in his arm. We were worried, and his wife and daughters were terrified, but gradually he pulled through.

By the third day after surgery, he was well enough to take sips of clear liquids (water, apple juice, ginger ale), up to one ounce every four hours. On my afternoon rounds, I asked him how the sips had gone down. "OK," he said. We began giving him four-ounce servings of Carnation Instant Breakfast for protein and modest calories. He could finish only half, and that took him an hour. It filled him up and, when it did, he felt a sharp, unpleasant pain. This was to be expected, Dr. Randall told him. It would be a few days before he was ready for solid food. But he was doing well. He no longer needed IV fluids. The pain from his wound was under control. And, after he'd had a short stay in a rehabilitation facility, we sent him home.

A couple of weeks later, I asked Dr. Randall how Caselli was getting on. "Just fine," the surgeon said. Although I had done a few of these cases with him, I had not seen how the patients progressed afterward. Would he really lose all that weight? I asked. And how much could he eat? Randall suggested that I see Caselli for myself. So one day that October, I gave him a call. He seemed happy to hear from me. "Come on by," he said. And after work that day, I did.

Vincent Caselli and his wife live in an unassuming saltbox house not far outside Boston. To get there, I took Route 1, past four ___in' Donuts, four pizzerias, three steak houses, two McDonald's, two Ground Rounds, a Taco Bell, a Friendly's, and an International House of Pancakes. (A familiar roadside vista, but that day it seemed a sad tour of our self-destructiveness.) I rang the doorbell, and a long minute passed. I heard a slow footfall coming toward the door, and Caselli, visibly winded, opened it. But he smiled broadly when he saw me, and gave my hand a warm squeeze. He led me—his hand on table, wall, doorjamb for support—to a seat at a breakfast table in his flowered-wallpaper kitchen.

I asked him how things were going. "Real good," he said. He had no more pain from the operation, the incision had healed, and, though it had been only three weeks, he'd already lost forty pounds. But, at three hundred and ninety, and still stretching his size 64 slacks and size XXXXXXL T-shirts (the largest he could find at the local big-and-tall store), he did not yet feel different. Sitting, he had to keep his legs apart to let his abdomen sag between them, and the weight of his body on the wooden chair forced him to shift every minute or two because his buttocks would fall asleep. Sweat rimmed the folds of his forehead and made his thin salt-and-pepper hair stick to his pate. His brown eyes were rheumy and had dark bags beneath them. He breathed with a disconcerting wheeze.

We talked about his arrival home from the hospital. The first solid food he had tried was a spoonful of scrambled eggs. Just that much made him so full it hurt, he said, really hurt, "like something was ripping," and he threw it back up. He was afraid that nothing solid would ever go down. But he gradually found that he could tolerate small amounts of soft foods—mashed potatoes, macaroni, even chicken if it was finely chopped and moist. Breads and dry meats, he found, got "stuck," and he'd have to put a finger down his throat and make himself vomit.

It troubled Caselli that things had come to this, but he had made peace with the need for it. "Last year or two, I'm in hell," he said. The battle had begun in his late twenties. "I always had some weight on me," he said. He was two hundred pounds at nineteen, when he married Teresa (as I'll call her), and a decade later he reached three hundred. He would diet and lose seventy-five pounds, then put a hundred back on. By 1985, he weighed four hundred pounds. On one diet, he got all the way down to a hundred and ninety. Then he shot back up again. "I must have gained and lost a thousand pounds," he told me. He developed high blood pressure, high cholesterol, and diabetes. His knees and his back ached all the time. He had only limited mobility. He used to get season tickets to Boston Bruins games, and go out regularly to the track at Seekonk every summer to see the auto racing. Years ago, he drove in races himself. Now he could barely walk to his pickup truck. He hadn't been on an airplane since 1983, and it had been two years since he had been to the second floor of his own house, because he couldn't negotiate the stairs. "Teresa bought a computer a year ago for her office upstairs, and I've never seen it," he told me. He had to move out of their bedroom, upstairs, to a small room off the kitchen. Unable to lie down, he had slept in a recliner ever since. Even so, he could doze only in snatches, because of sleep apnea, which is a common syndrome among the obese, thought to be related to excessive fat in the tongue and in the soft tissues of the upper airway. Every thirty minutes, his breathing would stop, and he'd wake up asphyxiating. He was perpetually exhausted.

There were other troubles, too, the kind that few people speak about. Good hygiene, he said, was nearly impossible. He could no longer stand up to urinate, and after moving his bowels he often had to shower in order to get clean. Skin folds would become chafed and red, and sometimes develop boils and infections. "Has it been a strain on your marriage?" I asked. "Sure," he said. "Sex life is nonexistent. I have real hopes for it." For him, though, the worst part was his diminishing ability to earn a livelihood.

Vincent Caselli's father had come to Boston from Italy in 1914 to work in construction. Before long, he had acquired five steam shovels and established his own firm. In the 1960s, Vince and his brother took over the business, and in 1979 Vince went into business for himself. He was skilled at operating heavy equipment—his specialty was running a Gradall, a thirty-ton, three-hundred-thousand-dollar hydraulic excavator—and he employed a team of men year-round to build roads and sidewalks. Eventually, he owned his own Gradall, a ten-wheel Mack dump truck, a backhoe, and a fleet of pickup trucks. But in the past three years he had become too big to operate the Gradall or keep up with the daily maintenance of the equipment. He had to run the business from his house, and pay others to do the heavy work; he enlisted a nephew to help manage the men and the contracts. Expenses rose, and because he could no longer make the rounds of city halls himself, he found contracts harder and harder to get. If it hadn't been for Teresa's job—she is the business manager for an assisted-living facility in Boston—they would have gone bankrupt.

Teresa, a pretty, freckled redhead (of, as it happens, fairly normal weight) had been pushing him for a long time to diet and exercise. He, too, wanted desperately to lose weight, but the task of controlling himself, day to day, meal to meal, seemed beyond him. "I'm a man of habits," he told me. "I'm very prone to habits." And eating, he said, was his worst habit. But, then, eating is everyone's habit. What was different about *his* habit? I asked. Well, the portions he took were too big, and he could never leave a crumb on his plate. If there was pasta left in the pot, he'd eat that, too. But why, I wanted to know. Was it just that he loved food? He pondered this question for a moment. It wasn't love, he decided. "Eating felt good instantaneously," he said, "but it only felt good instantaneously." Was it excessive hunger that drove him? "I was never hungry," he said.

As far as I could tell, Caselli ate for the same reasons that everyone eats: because food tasted good, because it was seven o'clock and time for dinner, because a nice meal had been set out on the table. And he stopped eating for the same reason everyone stops: because he was full and eating was no longer pleasurable. The main difference seemed to be that it took an unusual quantity of food to make him full. (He could eat a large pizza without blinking.) To lose weight, he faced the same difficult task that every dieter faces—to stop eating before he felt full, while the food still tasted good, and to exercise. These were things that he could do for a little while, and, with some reminding and coaching, for perhaps a bit longer, but they were not, he had found, things that he could do for long. "I am not strong," he said.

In early 1998, Caselli's internist sternly told him, "If you cannot take off this weight, we are going to have to do something drastic." And by this she meant surgery. She described the gastric-bypass operation to him and gave him Dr. Randall's number. To Caselli, it was out of the question. The idea of the procedure was troubling enough. No way could he put his business on hold for that. A year later, however, in the spring of 1999, he developed bad infections in both legs: as his weight increased, and varicosities appeared, the skin thinned and broke down, producing open, purulent ulcers. Despite fevers and searing pain, it was only after persistent coaxing from his wife that he finally agreed to see his doctor. The doctor diagnosed a serious case of cellulitis, and he spent a week in the hospital receiving intravenous antibiotics.

At the hospital, he was also given an ultrasound scan to check for blood clots in his legs. Afterward, a radiologist came to give him the results. "He says, 'You're a lucky guy,'" Caselli recounted. "I say, 'Did I win the lottery? Wha'd I do?' He says, 'You don't have blood clots, and I'm really surprised.' He says, 'I don't mean to break your bubble, but a guy like you, in the situation you're in, the odds are you're gonna have blood clots. That tells me you're a pretty healthy guy'"—but only, he went on, if Caselli did something about his weight.

A little later, the infectious-disease specialist came to see him. The specialist removed his bandages, examined his wounds, and wrapped them back up again. His legs were getting better, he said. But then he added one more thing. "'I'm going to tell you something,'" Caselli recalls the man saying. "'I've been reading your whole file—where you were, what you were, how you were. Now you're here and this is what's going on. You take that weight off—and I'm not telling you this to bust your ass, I'm *telling* you—you take that weight off and you're a very healthy guy. Your heart is good. Your lungs are good. You're strong.'"

"I took that seriously," Caselli said. "You know, there are two different doctors telling me this. They don't know me other than what they're reading from their records. They had no reason to tell me this. But they knew the weight was a problem. And if I could get it down . . ."

When he got home, he remained sick in bed for another two weeks. Meanwhile, his business collapsed. Contracts stopped coming in entirely, and he knew that when his men finished the existing jobs he would have to let them go. Teresa made an appointment for him to see Dr. Randall, and he went. Randall described the gastric-bypass operation and spoke with him frankly about the risks involved. There was a one-in-two-hundred chance of death and a one-in-ten chance of an untoward outcome, such as bleeding, infection, gastric ulceration, blood clots, or leakage into the abdomen. The doctor also told him that it would change how he ate forever. Unable to work, humiliated, ill, and in pain, Vincent Caselli decided that surgery was his only hope.

It is hard to contemplate the human appetite without wondering if we have any say over our lives at all. We believe in will—in the notion that we have a choice over such simple matters as whether to sit still or stand up, to talk or not talk, to have a slice of pie or not. Yet very few people, whether heavy or slim, can voluntarily reduce their weight for long. The history of weight-loss treatment is one of nearly unremitting failure. Whatever the regimen—liquid diets, high-protein diets, or grapefruit diets, the Zone, Atkins, or Dean Ornish diet—people lose weight quite readily, but they do not keep it off. A 1993 National Institutes of Health expert panel reviewed decades of diet studies and found that between 90 and 95 percent of people regained one-third to two-thirds of any weight lost within a year—and all of it within five years. Doctors have wired patients' jaws closed, inflated plastic balloons inside their stomachs, performed massive excisions of body fat, prescribed amphetamines and large amounts of thyroid hormone, even performed neurosurgery to destroy the hunger centers in the brain's hypothalamus—and still people do not keep the weight off. Jaw wiring, for example, can produce substantial weight loss, and patients who ask for the procedure are as motivated as they come; yet some still end up taking in enough liquid calories through their closed jaws to gain weight, and the others regain it once the wires are removed. We are a species that has evolved to survive starvation, not to resist abundance.

The one group of human beings that stands in exception to this doleful history of failure is, surprisingly, children. Nobody would argue that children have more self-control than adults; yet in four randomized studies of obese children between the ages of six and twelve, those who received simple behavioral teaching (weekly lessons for eight to twelve weeks, followed by monthly meetings for up to a year) ended up markedly less overweight ten years later than those who didn't; 30 percent were no longer obese. Apparently, children's appetites are malleable. Those of adults are not.

The revealing moment is the meal. There are at least two ways that humans can eat more than they ought to at a sitting. One is by eating slowly but steadily for far too long. This is what people with Prader-Willi syndrome do. Afflicted with a rare inherited dysfunction of the hypothalamus, they are incapable of experiencing satiety. And though they eat only half as quickly as most people, they do not stop. Unless their access to food is strictly controlled (some will eat garbage or pet food if they find nothing else), they become mortally obese.

The more common pattern, however, relies on rapid intake. Human beings are subject to what scientists call a "fat paradox." When food enters your stomach and duodenum (the upper portion of the small intestine), it triggers stretch receptors, protein receptors, and fat receptors that signal the hypothalamus to induce satiety. Nothing stimulates the reaction more quickly than fat. Even a small amount, once it reaches the duodenum, will cause a person to stop eating. Still we eat too much fat. How can this be? The reason is speed. It turns out that foods can trigger receptors in the mouth which get the hypothalamus to *accelerate* our intake—and, again, the most potent stimulant is fat. A little bit on the tongue, and the receptors push us to eat fast, before the gut signals shut us down. The tastier the food, the faster we eat—a phenomenon called "the appetizer effect." (This is accomplished, in case you were wondering, not by chewing faster but by chewing less. French researchers have discovered that, in order to eat more and eat it faster, people shorten their "chewing time"—they take fewer "chews per standard food unit" before swallowing. In other words, we gulp.)

Apparently, how heavy one becomes is determined, in part, by how the hypothalamus and the brain stem adjudicate the conflicting signals from the mouth and the gut. Some people feel full quite early in a meal; others, like Vincent Caselli, experience the appetizer effect for much longer. In the past several years, much has been discovered about the mechanisms of this control. We now know, for instance, that hormones, like leptin and neuropeptide Y, rise and fall with fat levels and adjust the appetite accordingly. But our knowledge of these mechanisms is still crude at best.

Consider a 1998 report concerning two men, "BR" and "RH," who suffered from profound amnesia. Like the protagonist in the movie *Memento*, they could carry on a coherent conversation with you, but, once they had been distracted, they recalled nothing from as recently as a minute before, not even that they were talking to you. (BR had had a bout of viral encephalitis; RH had had a severe seizure disorder for twenty years.) Paul Rozin, a professor of psychology at the University of Pennsylvania, thought of using them in an experiment that would explore the relationship between memory and eating. On three consecutive days, he and his team brought each subject his typical lunch (BR got meat loaf, barley soup, tomatoes, potatoes, beans, bread, butter, peaches, and tea; RH got veal parmigiana with pasta, string beans, juice, and apple crumb cake). Each day, BR ate all his lunch, and RH could not quite finish.

Their plates were then taken away. Ten to thirty minutes later, the researchers would reappear with the same meal. "Here's lunch," they would announce. The men ate just as much as before. Another ten to thirty minutes later, the researchers again appeared with the same meal. "Here's lunch," they would say, and again the men would eat. On a couple of occasions, the researchers even offered RH a fourth lunch. Only then did he decline, saying that his "stomach was a little tight." Stomach stretch receptors weren't completely ineffectual. Yet, in the absence of a memory of having eaten, social context alone—someone walking in with lunch—was enough to re-create appetite.

You can imagine forces in the brain vying to make you feel hungry or full. You have mouth receptors, smell receptors, visions of tiramisu pushing one way and gut receptors another. You have leptins and neuropeptides saying you have either too much fat stored or too little. And you have your own social and personal sense of whether eating more is a good idea. If one mechanism is thrown out of whack, there's trouble.

Given the complexity of appetite and our imperfect understanding of it, we shouldn't be surprised that appetite-altering drugs have had only meager success in making people eat less. (The drug combination of fenfluramine and phentermine, or "fen-phen," had the most success, but it was linked to heart valve abnormalities and was withdrawn from the market.) University researchers and pharmaceutical companies are searching intensively for a drug that will effectively treat serious obesity. So far, no such drug exists. Nonetheless, one treatment has been found to be effective, and, oddly enough, it turns out to be an operation.

At my hospital, there is a recovery room nurse who is forty-eight years old and just over five feet tall, with boyish sandy hair and an almost athletic physique. Over coffee one day at the hospital café, not long after my visit with Vincent Caselli, she revealed that she once weighed more than two hundred and fifty pounds. Carla (as I'll call her) explained that she had had gastric-bypass surgery some fifteen years ago.

She had been obese since she was five years old. She started going on diets and taking diet pills—laxatives, diuretics, amphetamines—in junior high school. "It was never a problem losing weight," she said. "It was a problem keeping it off." She remembers how upset she was when, on a trip with friends to Disneyland, she found that she couldn't fit through the entrance turnstile. At the age of thirty-three, she reached two hundred and sixty-five pounds. One day, accompanying her partner, a physician, to a New Orleans medical convention, she found that she was too short of breath to walk down Bourbon Street. For the first time, she said, "I became fearful for my life—not just the quality of it but the longevity of it."

That was 1985. Doctors were experimenting with radical obesity surgery, but there was dwindling enthusiasm for it. Two operations had held considerable promise. One, known as jejuno-ileal bypass— in which nearly all the small intestine was bypassed, so that only a minimum amount of food could be absorbed—turned out to be killing people. The other, stomach stapling, was proving to lose its effectiveness over time; people tended to adapt to the tiny stomach, eating densely caloric foods more and more frequently.

Working in the hospital, however, Carla heard encouraging reports about the gastric-bypass operation—stomach stapling plus a rerouting of the intestine so that food bypassed only the first meter of small intestine. She knew that the data about its success was still sketchy and that other operations had failed, and she took a year to decide. But the more she gained, the more convinced she became that she had to take the chance. In May of 1986, she went ahead and had the surgery.

"For the first time in my life, I experienced fullness," she told me. Six months after the operation, she was down to a hundred and eighty-five pounds. Six months after that, she weighed a hundred and thirty pounds. She lost so much weight that she had to have surgery to remove the aprons of skin that hung from her belly and thighs down to her knees. She was unrecognizable to anyone who had known her before, and even to herself. "I went to bars to see if I could get picked up—and I did," she said. "I always said no," she quickly added, laughing. "But I did it anyway."

The changes weren't just physical, though. She had slowly found herself to have a profound and unfamiliar sense of willpower over food. She no longer *had* to eat anything: "Whenever I eat, somewhere in the course of that time I end up asking myself, 'Is this good for you? Are you going to put on weight if you eat too much of this?' And I can just stop." The feeling baffled her. She knew, intellectually, that the surgery was why she no longer ate as much as she used to. Yet she felt as if she were choosing not to do it.

Studies report this to be a typical experience of successful gastric-bypass patients. "I do get hungry, but I tend to think about it more," another woman who had had the operation told me, and she described an internal dialogue very much like Carla's: "I ask myself, 'Do I really need this?' I watch myself." For many, this feeling of control extends beyond eating. They become more confident, even assertive—sometimes to the point of conflict. Divorce rates, for example, have been found to increase significantly after the surgery. Indeed, a few months after her operation, Carla and her partner broke up.

Carla's dramatic weight loss has proved to be no aberration. Published case series now show that most patients undergoing gastric bypass lose at least two-thirds of their excess weight (generally more than a hundred pounds) within a year. They keep it off, too: ten-year follow-up studies find an average regain of only ten to twenty pounds. And the health benefits are striking: patients are less likely to have heart failure, asthma, or arthritis; most remarkable of all, 80 percent of those with diabetes are completely cured of it.

I stopped in to see Vincent Caselli one morning in January of 2000, about four months after his operation. He didn't quite spring to the door, but he wasn't winded this time. The bags under his eyes had shrunk. His face was more defined. Although his midriff was vast, it seemed smaller, less of a sack.

He told me that he weighed three hundred and forty-eight pounds—still far too much for a man who was only five feet seven inches tall, but ninety pounds less than he weighed on the operating table. And it had already made a difference in his life. Back in October, he told me, he missed his youngest daughter's wedding because he couldn't manage the walking required to get to the church. But by December he had lost enough weight to resume going to his East Dedham garage every morning. "Yesterday, I unloaded three tires off the truck," he said. "For me to do that three months ago? There's no way." He had climbed the stairs of his house for the first time since 1997. "One day around Christmastime, I say to myself, 'Let me try this. I gotta try this.' I went very slow, one foot at a time." The second floor was nearly unrecognizable to him. The bathroom had been renovated since he last saw it, and Teresa had, naturally, taken over the bedroom, including the closets. He would move back up eventually, he said, though it might be a while. He still had to sleep sitting up in a recliner, but he was sleeping in four-hour stretches now—"Thank God," he said. His diabetes was gone. And although he was still unable to stand up longer than twenty minutes, his leg ulcers were gone, too. He lifted his pants legs to show me. I noticed that he was wearing regular Red Wing work boots—in the past, he had to cut slits along the sides of his shoes in order to fit into them.

"I've got to lose at least another hundred pounds," he said. He wanted to be able to work, pick up his grandchildren, buy clothes off the rack at Filene's, go places without having to ask himself, "Are there stairs? Will I fit in the seats? Will I run out of breath?" He was still eating like a bird. The previous day, he'd had nothing all morning, a morsel of chicken with some cooked carrots and a small roast potato for lunch, and for dinner one fried shrimp, one teriyaki chicken strip, and two forkfuls of chicken-and-vegetable lo mein from a Chinese restaurant. He was starting up the business again, and, he told me, he'd gone out for a business lunch one day recently. It was at a new restaurant in Hyde Park—"beautiful," he said—and he couldn't help ordering a giant burger and a plate of fries. Just two bites into the burger, though, he had to stop. "One of the fellas says to me, 'Is that all you're going to eat?' And I say, 'I can't eat any more.' 'Really?' I say, 'Yeah, I can't eat any more. That's the truth.'"

I noticed, however, that the way he spoke about eating was not the way Carla had spoken. He did not speak of stopping because he wanted to. He spoke of stopping because he had to. You want to eat more, he explained, but "you start to get that feeling in your insides that one more bite is going to push you over the top." Still, he often took that bite. Overcome by waves of nausea, pain, and bloating— the so-called dumping syndrome—he'd have to vomit. If there was a way to eat more, he would. This scared him, he admitted. "It's not right," he said.

Three months later, in April, Vince invited me and my son to stop by his garage in East Dedham. Walker was four years old then and, as Vince remembered my once saying, fascinated with all things mechanical. So on my Saturday off, we went. As we pulled into the gravel lot, Walker was fairly zizzing with excitement. The garage was cavernous, barnlike, with a two-story garage door and metal walls painted yellow. Outside, it was an unusually warm spring morning, but inside the air was cool. Our footsteps echoed on the concrete floor. Vince and a buddy of his, a fellow heavy-equipment contractor I'll call Danny, were sitting on metal folding chairs in a sliver of sunlight, puffing fat Honduran cigars, silently enjoying the day. Both rose to greet us. Vince introduced me as "one of the doctors who did my stomach operation," and I introduced Walker, who shook hands all around but saw only the big trucks. Vince lifted him up into the driver's seat of a front-end loader backhoe in one corner of the garage and let him play with the knobs and controls. Then we went over to Vince's beloved Gradall, a handsome tank of a machine, wide as a county road, painted yield-sign yellow, with shiny black tires that came up to my chest and the name of his company emblazoned in curlicue script along its flanks. On the chassis, six feet off the ground, was a glass-enclosed cab and a thirty-foot tele-scoping boom on a three-hundred-and-sixty-degree swivel. We hoisted Walker up into the cab and he stood there awhile, high above us, pulling levers and pressing pedals, giddy and scared all at once.

I asked Vince how his business was going. Not well, he said. Except for a few jobs in late winter plowing snow for the city in his pickup truck, he had brought in no income since the previous August. He'd had to sell two of his three pickups, his Mack dump truck, and most of the small equipment for road building. Danny came to his defense. "Well, he's been out of action," he said. "And you see we're just coming into the summer season. It's a seasonal business." But we all knew that wasn't the issue.

Vince told me that he weighed about three hundred and twenty pounds. This was about thirty pounds less than when I had last seen him, and he was proud of that. "He don't eat," Danny said. "He eats half of what I eat." But Vince was still unable to climb up into the Gradall and operate it. And he was beginning to wonder whether that would ever change. The rate of weight loss was slowing down, and he noticed that he was able to eat more. Before, he could eat only a couple of bites of a burger, but now he could sometimes eat half of one. And he still found himself eating more than he could handle. "Last week, Danny and this other fellow, we had to do some business," he said. "We had Chinese food. Lots of days, I don't eat the right stuff—I try to do what I can do, but I ate a little bit too much. I had to bring Danny back to Boston College, and before I left the parking lot there I just couldn't take it anymore. I had to vomit.

"I'm finding that I'm getting back into that pattern where I've always got to eat," he went on. His gut still stopped him, but he was worried. What if one day it didn't? He had heard about people whose staples gave way, returning their stomach to its original size, or who managed to put the weight back on in some other way.

I tried to reassure him. I told him what I knew Dr. Randall had already told him during a recent appointment: that a small increase in the capacity of his stomach pouch was to be expected, and that what he was experiencing seemed normal. But could something worse happen? I didn't want to say.

Among the gastric-bypass patients I had talked with was a man whose story remains a warning and a mystery to me. He was forty-two years old, married, and had two daughters, both of whom were single mothers with babies and still lived at home, and he had been the senior computer-systems manager for a large local company. At the age of thirty-eight, he had had to retire and go on disability because his weight—which had been above three hundred pounds since high school—had increased to more than four hundred and fifty pounds and was causing unmanageable back pain. He was soon confined to his home. He could not walk half a block. He could stand for only brief periods. He went out, on average, once a week, usually for medical appointments. In December 1998, he had a gastric bypass. By June of the following year, he had lost a hundred pounds.

Then, as he put it, "I started eating again." Pizzas. Boxes of sugar cookies. Packages of doughnuts. He found it hard to say how, exactly. His stomach was still tiny and admitted only a small amount of food at a time, and he experienced the severe nausea and pain that gastric-bypass patients get whenever they eat sweet or rich things. Yet his drive was stronger than ever. "I'd eat right through pain—even to the point of throwing up," he told me. "If I threw up, it was just room for more. I would eat straight through the day." He did not pass a waking hour without eating something. "I'd just shut the bedroom door. The kids would be screaming. The babes would be crying. My wife would be at work. And I would be eating." His weight returned to four hundred and fifty pounds, and then more. The surgery had failed. And his life had been shrunk to the needs of pure appetite.

He is among the 5 to 20 percent of patients—the published reports conflict on the exact number—who regain weight despite gastric-bypass surgery. (When we spoke, he had recently submitted to another, more radical gastric bypass, in the desperate hope that something would work.) In these failures, one begins to grasp the depth of the power that one is up against. An operation that makes overeating both extremely difficult and extremely unpleasant—which, for more than 80 percent of patients, is finally sufficient to cause appetite to surrender and be transformed—can sometimes be defeated after all. Studies have yet to uncover a single consistent risk factor for this outcome. It could, apparently, happen to anyone.

Several months passed before I saw Vince Caselli again. Winter came, and I called him to see how he was doing. He said he was well, and I did not press for details. When we talked about getting together, though, he mentioned that it might be fun to go see a Boston Bruins game together, and my ears pricked up. Perhaps he *was* doing well.

A few days later, he picked me up at the hospital in his rumbling six-wheel Dodge Ram. For the first time since I'd met him, he looked almost small in that outsize truck. He was down to about two hundred and fifty pounds. "I'm still no Gregory Peck," he said, but he was now one of the crowd—chubby, in an ordinary way. The rolls beneath his chin were gone. His face had a shape. His middle no longer rested between his legs. And, almost a year and a half after the surgery, he was still losing weight. At the FleetCenter, where the Bruins play, he walked up the escalator without getting winded. Our tickets were taken at the gate—the Bruins were playing the Pittsburgh Penguins—and we walked through the turnstiles. Suddenly, he stopped. "Look at that," he exclaimed. "I went right through, no problem. I never would have made it through there before." It was the first time he'd gone to an event like this in years.

We took our seats about two dozen rows up from the ice, and he laughed a little about how easily he fit. The seats were as tight as coach class, but he was quite comfortable. (I, with my long legs, was the one who had trouble finding room.) Vince was right at home here. He had been a hockey fan his whole life, and could supply me with all the details: the Penguins' goalie Garth Snow was a local boy, from Wrentham, and a friend of one of Vince's cousins; Joe Thornton and Jason Allison were the Bruins' best forwards, but neither could hold a candle to the Penguins' Mario Lemieux. There were nearly twenty thousand people at the game, but within ten minutes Vince had found a friend from his barbershop sitting just a few rows away.

The Bruins won, and we left cheered and buzzing. Afterward, we went out to dinner at a grill near the hospital. Vince told me that his business was finally up and running. He could operate the Gradall without difficulty, and he'd had full-time Gradall work for the past three months. He was even thinking of buying a new model. At home, he had moved back upstairs. He and Teresa had taken a vacation in the Adirondacks; they were going out evenings, and visiting their grandchildren.

I asked him what had changed since I saw him the previous spring. He could not say precisely, but he gave me an example. "I used to love Italian cookies, and I still do," he said. A year ago, he would have eaten to the point of nausea. "But now they're, I don't know, they're too sweet. I eat one now, and after one or two bites I just don't want it." It was the same with pasta, which had always been a problem for him. "Now I can have a taste and I'm satisfied."

Partly, it appeared that his taste in food had changed. He pointed to the nachos and Buffalo wings and hamburgers on the menu, and said that, to his surprise, he no longer felt like eating any of them. "It seems like I lean toward protein and vegetables nowadays," he said, and he ordered a chicken Caesar salad. But he also no longer felt the need to stuff himself. "I used to be real reluctant to push food away," he told me. "Now it's just—it's different." But when did this happen? And how? He shook his head. "I wish I could pinpoint it for you," he said. He paused to consider. "As a human, you adjust to conditions. You don't think you are. But you are."

These days, it isn't the failure of obesity surgery that is prompting concerns but its success. For a long time it was something of a bastard child in respectable surgical circles. Bariatric surgeons—as obesity surgery specialists are called—faced widespread skepticism about the wisdom of forging ahead with such a radical operation when so many previous versions had failed, and there was sometimes fierce resistance to their even presenting their results at the top surgical conferences. They sensed the contempt other surgeons had for their patients (who were regarded as having an emotional, even moral, problem) and often for them.

This has all changed now. The American College of Surgeons recently recognized bariatric surgery as an accepted specialty. The National Institutes of Health issued a consensus statement endorsing gastric-bypass surgery as the only known effective therapy for morbid obesity, one able to produce long-term weight loss and improvement in health. And most insurers have agreed to pay for it.

Physicians have gone from scorning it to encouraging, sometimes imploring, their severely overweight patients to undergo a gastric-bypass operation. And that's not a small number of patients. More than five million adult Americans meet the strict definition of morbid obesity. (Their "body mass index"—that is, their weight in kilograms divided by the square of their height in meters—is forty or more, which for an average man is roughly a hundred pounds or more overweight.) Ten million more weigh just under the mark but may nevertheless have obesity-related health problems that are serious enough to warrant the surgery. There are ten times as many candidates for obesity surgery right now as there are for heart-bypass surgery in a year. So many patients are seeking the procedure that established surgeons cannot keep up with the demand. The American Society of Bariatric Surgery has only five hundred members nationwide who perform gastric-bypass operations, and their waiting lists are typically months long. Hence the too familiar troubles associated with new and lucrative surgical techniques (the fee can be as much as twenty thousand dollars): newcomers are stampeding to the field, including many who have proper training but have not yet mastered the procedure, and others who have no training at all. Complicating matters further, individual surgeons are promoting a slew of variations on the standard operation which haven't been fully researched—the "duodenal switch," the "long limb" bypass, the laparoscopic bypass. And a few surgeons are pursuing new populations, such as adolescents and people who are only moderately obese.

Perhaps what's most unsettling about the soaring popularity of gastric-bypass surgery, however, is simply the world that surrounds it. Ours is a culture in which fatness is seen as tantamount to failure, and get-thin-quick promises—whatever the risks—can have an irresistible allure. Doctors may recommend the operation out of concern for their patients' health, but the stigma of obesity is clearly what drives many patients to the operating room. "How can you let yourself look like that?" is often society's sneering, unspoken question, and sometimes its spoken one as well. (Caselli told me of strangers coming up to him on the street and asking him precisely this.) Women suffer even more than men from the social sanction, and it's no accident that seven times as many women as men have had the operation. (Women are only an eighth more likely to be obese.)

Indeed, deciding *not* to undergo the surgery, if you qualify, is at risk of being considered the unreasonable thing to do. A three-hundred-fifty-pound woman who did not want the operation told me of doctors browbeating her for her choice. And I have learned of at least one patient with heart disease being refused treatment by a doctor unless she had a gastric bypass. If you don't have the surgery, you will die, some doctors tell their patients. But we actually do not know this. Despite the striking improvements in weight and health, studies have not yet proved a corresponding reduction in mortality.

There are legitimate grounds for being wary of the procedure. As Paul Ernsberger, an obesity researcher at Case Western Reserve University, pointed out to me, many patients undergoing gastric bypass are in their twenties and thirties. "But is this really going to be effective and worthwhile over a forty-year span?" he asked. "No one can say." He was concerned about the possible long-term effects of nutritional deficiencies (for which patients are instructed to take a daily multivitamin). And he was concerned about evidence from rats that raises the possibility of an increased risk of bowel cancer.

We want progress in medicine to be clear and unequivocal, but of course it rarely is. Every new treatment has gaping unknowns—for both patients and society—and it can be hard to decide what to do about them. Perhaps a simpler, less radical operation will prove effective for obesity. Perhaps the long-sought satiety pill will be found. Nevertheless, the gastric bypass is the one thing we have now that works. Not all the questions have been answered, but there are more than a decade of studies behind it. And so we forge ahead. Hospitals everywhere are constructing obesity-surgery centers, ordering reinforced operating tables, training surgeons and staff. At the same time, everyone expects that, one day, something new and better will be discovered that will make what we're now doing obsolete.

Across from me, in our booth at the grill, Vince Caselli pushed his chicken Caesar salad aside only half eaten. "No taste for it," he said, and he told me he was grateful for that. He had no regrets about the operation. It had given him his life back, he said. But, after one more round of drinks and with the hour growing late, it was clear that he still felt uneasy.

"I had a serious problem and I had to take serious measures," he said. "I think I had the best technology that is available at this point. But I do get concerned: Is this going to last my whole life? Someday, am I going to be right back to square one—or worse?" He fell silent for a moment, gazing into his glass. Then he looked up, his eyes clear. "Well, that's the cards that God gave me. I can't worry about stuff I can't control."

Part III

Uncertainty

Final Cut

Your patient is dead; the family is gathered. And there is one last thing that you have to ask about: the autopsy. How should you go about it? You could do it offhandedly, as if it were the most ordinary thing in the world: "Shall we do an autopsy, then?" Or you could be firm, use your Sergeant Joe Friday voice: "Unless you have strong objections, we will need to do an autopsy, ma'am." Or you could take yourself out of it: "I am sorry, but they require me to ask, Do you want an autopsy done?"

What you can't be nowadays is mealymouthed about it. I once took care of a woman in her eighties who had given up her driver's license only to get hit by a car—driven by someone even older—while she was walking to a bus stop. She sustained a depressed skull fracture and cerebral bleeding, and, despite surgery, she died a few days later. So, on the spring afternoon after the patient took her last breath, I stood beside her and bowed my head with the tearful family. Then, as delicately as I could—not even using the awful word—I said, "If it's all right, we'd like to do an examination to confirm the cause of death."

"An *autopsy*?" a nephew said, horrified. He looked at me as if I were a buzzard circling his aunt's body. "Hasn't she been through enough?"

The autopsy is in a precarious state these days. A generation ago, it was routine; now it has become a rarity. Human beings have never quite become comfortable with the idea of having their bodies cut open after they die. Even for a surgeon, the sense of violation is inescapable.

Not long ago, I went to observe the dissection of a thirty-eight-year-old woman I had taken care of who had died after a long struggle with heart disease. The dissecting room was in the sub-basement, past the laundry and a loading dock, behind an unmarked metal door. It had high ceilings, peeling paint, and a brown tiled floor that sloped down to a central drain. There was a Bunsen burner on a countertop, and an old-style grocer's hanging scale, with a big clock-face red-arrow gauge and a pan underneath, for weighing organs. On shelves all around the room there were gray portions of brain, bowel, and other organs soaking in formalin in Tupperware-like containers. The facility seemed run-down, chintzy, low-tech. On a rickety gurney in the corner was my patient, sprawled out, completely naked. The autopsy team was just beginning its work.

Surgical procedures can be grisly, but dissections are somehow worse. In even the most gruesome operations—skin grafting, amputations—surgeons maintain some tenderness and aestheticism toward their work. We know that the bodies we cut still pulse with life, and that these are people who will wake again. But in the dissecting room, where the person is gone and only the shell remains, you naturally find little delicacy, and the difference is visible in the smallest details. There is, for example, the simple matter of how a body is moved from gurney to table. In the operating room, we follow a careful, elaborate procedure for the unconscious patient, involving a canvas-sleeved rolling board and several gentle movements. We don't want so much as a bruise. Down here, by contrast, someone grabbed my patient's arm, another person a leg, and they just yanked. When her skin stuck to the stainless-steel dissecting table, they had to wet her and the table down with a hose before they could pull her the rest of the way.

The young pathologist for the case stood on the sidelines and let a pathology assistant take the knife. Like many of her colleagues, the pathologist had not been drawn to her field by autopsies but by the high-tech detective work that she got to do on tissue from living patients. She was happy to leave the dissection to the assistant, who had more experience at it anyway.

The assistant was a tall, slender woman of around thirty with straight sandy-brown hair. She was wearing the full protective garb of mask, face shield, gloves, and blue plastic gown. Once the body was on the table, she placed a six-inch metal block under the back, between the shoulder blades, so that the head fell back and the chest arched up. Then she took a scalpel in her hand, a big No. 6 blade, and made a huge Y-shaped incision that came down diagonally from each shoulder, curving slightly around each breast before reaching the midline, and then continued down the abdomen to the pubis.

Surgeons get used to the opening of bodies. It is easy to detach yourself from the person on the table and become absorbed by the details of method and anatomy. Nevertheless, I couldn't help wincing as she did her work: she was holding the scalpel like a pen, which forced her to cut slowly and jaggedly with the tip of the blade. Surgeons are taught to stand straight and parallel to their incision, hold the knife between the thumb and four fingers, like a violin bow, and draw the belly of the blade through the skin in a single, smooth slice to the exact depth desired. The assistant was practically sawing her way through my patient.

From there, the evisceration was swift. The assistant flayed back the skin flaps. With an electric saw, she cut through the exposed ribs along both sides. Then she lifted the rib cage as if it were the hood of a car, opened the abdomen, and removed all the major organs—including the heart, the lungs, the liver, the bowels, and the kidneys. Then the skull was sawed open, and the brain, too, was removed. Meanwhile, the pathologist was at a back table, weighing and examining everything, and preparing samples for microscopy and thorough testing.

For all this, however, I had to admit: the patient came out looking remarkably undisturbed. The assistant had followed the usual procedure and kept the skull incision behind the woman's ears, where it was completely hidden by her hair. She had also taken care to close the chest and abdomen neatly, sewing the incision tight with weaved seven-cord thread. My patient seemed much the same as before, except now a little collapsed in the middle. (The standard consent allows the hospital to keep the organs for testing and research. This common and long-established practice has caused huge controversy in Britain—the media have branded it "organ stripping"—but in America it remains generally accepted.) Most families, in fact, still have open-casket funerals after autopsies. Morticians employ fillers to restore a corpse's shape, and when they're done you cannot tell that an autopsy has been performed.

Still, when it is time to ask for a family's permission to do such a thing, the images weigh on everyone's mind—not least the doctor's. You strive to achieve a cool, dispassionate attitude toward these matters. But doubts nevertheless creep in.

One of the first patients for whom I was expected to request an autopsy was a seventy-five-year-old retired New England doctor who died one winter night while I was with him. Herodotus Sykes (not his real name, but not unlike it, either) had been rushed to the hospital with an infected, rupturing abdominal aortic aneurysm and taken to emergency surgery. He survived it, and recovered steadily until, eighteen days later, his blood pressure dropped alarmingly and blood began to pour from a drainage tube in his abdomen. "The aortic stump must have blown out," his surgeon said. Residual infection must have weakened the suture line where the infected aorta had been removed. We could have operated again, but the patient's chances were poor, and his surgeon didn't think he would be willing to take any more.

He was right. No more surgery, Sykes told me. He'd been through enough. We called Mrs. Sykes, who was staying with a friend about two hours away, and she set out for the hospital.

It was about midnight. I sat with him as he lay silent and bleeding, his arms slack at his sides, his eyes without fear. I imagined his wife out on the Mass Pike, frantic, helpless, with six lanes, virtually empty at that hour, stretching far ahead.

Sykes held on, and at 2:15 A.M. his wife arrived. She turned ashen at the sight of him, but she steadied herself. She gently took his hand in hers. She squeezed, and he squeezed back. I left them to themselves.

At 2:45, the nurse called me in. I listened with my stethoscope, then turned to Mrs. Sykes and told her that he was gone. She had her husband's Yankee reserve, but she broke into quiet tears, weeping into her hands, and seemed suddenly frail and small. A friend who had come with her soon appeared, took her by the arm, and led her out of the room.

We are instructed to request an autopsy on everyone as a means of confirming the cause of death and catching our mistakes. And this was the moment I was supposed to ask—with the wife despondent and reeling with shock. But surely, I began to think, here was a case in which an autopsy would be pointless. We knew what had happened—a persistent infection, a rupture. We were sure of it. What would cutting the man apart accomplish?

And so I let Mrs. Sykes go. I could have caught her as she walked through the ICU's double doors. Or even called her on the phone later. But I never did.

Such reasoning, it appears, has become commonplace in medicine. Doctors are seeking so few autopsies that in recent years the *Journal of the American Medical Association* has twice felt the need to declare "war on the nonautopsy." According to the most recent statistics available, autopsies have been done in fewer than 10 percent of deaths; many hospitals do none. This is a dramatic turnabout.

Through much of the twentieth century, doctors diligently obtained autopsies in the majority of all deaths—and it had taken centuries to reach this point. As Kenneth Iserson recounts in his fascinating almanac, *Death to Dust*, physicians have performed autopsies for more than two thousand years. But for most of history they were rarely performed. If religions permitted them at all—Islam, Shinto, orthodox Judaism, and the Greek Orthodox Church still frown on them—it was generally only for legal purposes. The Roman physician Antistius performed one of the earliest forensic examinations on record, in 44 B.C., on Julius Caesar, documenting twenty-three wounds, including a final, fatal stab to the chest. In 1410, the Catholic Church itself ordered an autopsy—on Pope Alexander V, to determine whether his successor had poisoned him. No evidence of this was apparently found.

The first documented postmortem examination in the New World was actually done for religious reasons, though. It was performed on July 19, 1533, on the island of Española (now the Dominican Republic), upon conjoined female twins connected at the lower chest, to determine if they had one soul or two. The twins had been born alive, and a priest had baptized them as two separate souls. A disagreement subsequently ensued about whether he was right to have done so, and when the "double monster" died at eight days of age an autopsy was ordered to settle the issue. A surgeon, one Johan Camacho, found two virtually complete sets of internal organs, and it was decided that two souls had lived and died.

Even in the nineteenth century, however, long after church strictures had loosened, people in the West seldom allowed doctors to autopsy their family members for medical purposes. As a result, the practice was largely clandestine. Some doctors went ahead and autopsied hospital patients immediately after death, before relatives could turn up to object. Others waited until burial and then robbed the graves, either personally or through accomplices, an activity that continued into the twentieth century. To deter such autopsies, some families would post nighttime guards at the grave site—hence the term "graveyard shift." Others placed heavy stones on the coffins. In 1878, one company in Columbus, Ohio, even sold "torpedo coffins," equipped with pipe bombs rigged to blow up if they were tampered with. Yet doctors remained undeterred. Ambrose Bierce's *The Devil's Dictionary*, published in 1906, defined "grave" as "a place in which the dead are laid to await the coming of the medical student."

By the turn of the twentieth century, however, prominent physicians such as Rudolf Virchow in Berlin, Karl Rokitansky in Vienna, and William Osler in Baltimore began to win popular support for the practice of autopsy. They defended it as a tool of discovery, one that had already been used to identify the cause of tuberculosis, reveal how to treat appendicitis, and establish the existence of Alzheimer's disease. They also showed that autopsies prevented errors—that without them doctors could not know when their diagnoses were incorrect. Moreover, most deaths were a mystery then, and perhaps what clinched the argument was the notion that autopsies could provide families with answers—give the story of a loved one's life a comprehensible ending. Once doctors had insured a dignified and respectful dissection at the hospital, public opinion turned. With time, doctors who did *not* obtain autopsies were viewed with suspicion. By the end of the Second World War, the autopsy was firmly established as a routine part of death in Europe and North America.

So what accounts for its decline? In truth, it's not because families refuse—to judge from recent studies, they still grant that permission up to 80 percent of the time. Instead, doctors, once so eager to perform autopsies that they stole bodies, have simply stopped asking. Some people ascribe this to shady motives. It has been said that hospitals are trying to save money by avoiding autopsies, since insurers don't pay for them, or that doctors avoid them in order to cover up evidence of malpractice. And yet autopsies lost money and uncovered malpractice when they were popular, too.

Instead, I suspect, what discourages autopsies is medicine's twenty-first-century, tall-in-the-saddle confidence. When I failed to ask Mrs. Sykes whether we could autopsy her husband, it was not because of the expense, or because I feared that the autopsy would uncover an error. It was the opposite: I didn't see much likelihood that an error would be found. Today, we have MRI scans, ultrasound, nuclear medicine, molecular testing, and much more. When somebody dies, we already know why. We don't need an autopsy to find out.

Or so I thought. Then I had a patient who changed my mind.

He was in his sixties, whiskered and cheerful, a former engineer who had found success in retirement as an artist. I will call him Mr. Jolly, because that's what he was. He was also what we call a vasculopath—he did not seem to have an undiseased artery in him. Whether because of his diet or his genes or the fact that he used to smoke, he had had, in the previous decade, one heart attack, two abdominal aortic aneurysm repairs, four bypass operations to keep blood flowing past blockages in his leg arteries, and several balloon procedures to keep hardened arteries open. Still, I never knew him to take a dark view of his lot. "Well, you can't get miserable about it," he'd say. He had wonderful children. He had beautiful grandchildren. "But, aargh, the wife," he'd go on. She would be sitting right there at the bedside and would roll her eyes, and he'd break into a grin.

Mr. Jolly had come into the hospital for treatment of a wound infection in his legs. But he soon developed congestive heart failure, causing fluid to back up into his lungs. Breathing became steadily harder for him, until we had to put him in the ICU, intubate him, and place him on a ventilator. A two-day admission turned into two weeks. With a regimen of diuretics and a change in heart medications, however, his heart failure reversed, and his lungs recovered. And one bright Sunday morning he was reclining in bed, breathing on his own, watching the morning shows on the TV set that hung from the ceiling. "You're doing marvelously," I said. I told him we would transfer him out of intensive care by the afternoon. He would probably be home in a couple of days.

Two hours later, a code-blue emergency call went out on the overhead speakers. When I got to the ICU and saw the nurse hunched over Mr. Jolly, doing chest compressions, I blurted out an angry curse. He'd been fine, the nurse explained, just watching TV, when suddenly he sat upright with a look of shock and then fell back, unresponsive. At first, he was asystolic—no heart rhythm on the monitor—and then the rhythm came back, but he had no pulse. A crowd of staffers set to work. I had him intubated, gave him fluids and epinephrine, had someone call the attending surgeon at home, someone else check the morning lab test results. An X-ray technician shot a portable chest film.

I mentally ran through possible causes. There were not many. A collapsed lung, but I heard good breath sounds with my stethoscope, and when his X ray came back the lungs looked fine. A massive blood loss, but his abdomen wasn't swelling, and his decline happened so quickly that bleeding just didn't make sense. Extreme acidity of the blood could do it, but his lab tests were fine. Then there was cardiac tamponade—bleeding into the sac that contains the heart. I took a six-inch spinal needle on a syringe, pushed it through the skin below the breastbone, and advanced it to the heart sac. I found no bleeding. That left only one possibility: a pulmonary embolism—a blood clot that flips into the lung and instantly wedges off all blood flow. And nothing could be done about that.

I went out and spoke to the attending surgeon by phone and then to the chief resident, who had just arrived. An embolism was the only logical explanation, they agreed. I went back into the room and stopped the code. "Time of death: 10:23 A.M.," I announced. I phoned his wife at home, told her that things had taken a turn for the worse, and asked her to come in.

This shouldn't have happened; I was sure of it. I scanned the records for clues. Then I found one. In a lab test done the day before, the patient's clotting had seemed slow, which wasn't serious, but an ICU physician had decided to correct it with vitamin K. A frequent side effect of vitamin K is blood clots. I was furious. Giving the vitamin was completely unnecessary—just fixing a number on a lab test. Both the chief resident and I lit into the physician. We all but accused him of killing the patient.

When Mrs. Jolly arrived, we took her to a family room where it was quiet and calm. I could see from her face that she'd already surmised the worst. His heart had stopped suddenly, we told her, because of a pulmonary embolism. We said the medicines we gave him may have contributed to it. I took her in to see him and left her with him. After a while, she came out, her hands trembling and her face stained with tears. Then, remarkably, she thanked us. We had kept him for her all these years, she said. Maybe so, but neither of us felt any pride about what had just happened.

I asked her the required question. I told her that we wanted to perform an autopsy and needed her permission. We thought we already knew what had happened, but an autopsy would confirm it, I said. She considered my request for a moment. If an autopsy would help us, she finally said, then we could do it. I said, as I was supposed to, that it would. I wasn't sure I believed it.

I wasn't assigned to the operating room the following morning, so I went down to observe the autopsy. When I arrived, Mr. Jolly was already laid out on the dissecting table, his arms splayed, skin flayed back, chest exposed, abdomen open. I put on a gown, gloves, and a mask, and went up close. The assistant began buzzing through the ribs on the left side with the electric saw, and immediately blood started seeping out, as dark and viscous as crankcase oil. Puzzled, I helped him lift open the rib cage. The left side of the chest was full of blood. I felt along the pulmonary arteries for a hardened, embolized clot, but there was none. He hadn't had an embolism after all. We suctioned out three liters of blood, lifted the left lung, and the answer appeared before our eyes. The thoracic aorta was almost three times larger than it should have been, and there was a half-inch hole in it. The man had ruptured an aortic aneurysm and had bled to death almost instantly.

In the days afterward, I apologized to the physician I'd reamed out over the vitamin, and pondered how we had managed to miss the diagnosis. I looked through the patient's old X rays and now saw a shadowy outline of what must have been his aneurysm. But none of us, not even the radiologists, had caught it. Even if we had caught it, we wouldn't have dared to do anything about it until weeks after treating his infection and heart failure, and that would have been too late. It disturbed me, however, to have felt so confident about what had happened that day and to have been so wrong.

The most perplexing thing was his final chest X ray, the one we had taken during the code blue. With all that blood filling the chest, I should have seen at least a haze over the left side. But when I pulled the film out to look again, there was nothing.

How often do autopsies turn up a major misdiagnosis in the cause of death? I would have guessed this happened rarely, in 1 or 2 percent of cases at most. According to three studies done in 1998 and 1999, however, the figure is about 40 percent. A large review of autopsy studies concluded that in about a third of the misdiagnoses the patients would have been expected to live if proper treatment had been administered. George Lundberg, a pathologist and former editor of the *Journal of the American Medical Association*, has done more than anyone to call attention to these figures. He points out the most surprising fact of all: the rates at which misdiagnosis is detected in autopsy studies have not improved since at least 1938.

With all the recent advances in imaging and diagnostics, it's hard to accept that we not only get the diagnosis wrong in two out of five of our patients who die but that we have also failed to improve over time. To see if this could really be true, doctors at Harvard put together a simple study. They went back into their hospital records to see how often autopsies picked up missed diagnoses in 1960 and 1970, before the advent of CT, ultrasound, nuclear scanning, and other technologies, and then in 1980, after those technologies became widely used. The researchers found no improvement. Regardless of the decade, physicians missed a quarter of fatal infections, a third of heart attacks, and almost two-thirds of pulmonary emboli in their patients who died.

In most cases, it wasn't technology that failed. Rather, the physicians did not consider the correct diagnosis in the first place. The perfect test or scan may have been available, but the physicians never ordered it.

In a 1976 essay, the philosophers Samuel Gorovitz and Alasdair MacIntyre explored the nature of fallibility. Why would a meteorologist, say, fail to correctly predict where a hurricane was going to make landfall? They saw three possible reasons. One was ignorance: perhaps science affords only a limited understanding of how hurricanes behave. A second reason was ineptitude: the knowledge is available, but the weatherman fails to apply it correctly. Both of these are surmountable sources of error. We believe that science will overcome ignorance, and that training and technology will overcome ineptitude. The third possible cause of error the philosophers posited, however, was an insurmountable kind, one they termed "necessary fallibility."

There may be some kinds of knowledge that science and technology will never deliver, Gorovitz and MacIntyre argued. When we ask science to move beyond explaining how things (say, hurricanes) generally behave to predicting exactly how a particular thing (say, Thursday's storm off the South Carolina coast) will behave, we may be asking it to do more than it can. No hurricane is quite like any other hurricane. Although all hurricanes follow predictable laws of behavior, each one is continuously shaped by myriad uncontrollable, accidental factors in the environment. To say precisely how one specific hurricane will behave would require a complete understanding of the world in all its particulars—in other words, omniscience.

It's not that it's impossible to predict anything; plenty of things are completely predictable. Gorovitz and MacIntyre give the example of a random ice cube in a fire. Ice cubes are so simple and so alike that you can predict with complete assurance that the ice cube will melt. But when it comes to inferring exactly what is going on in a particular person, are people more like ice cubes or like hurricanes?

Right now, at about midnight, I am seeing a patient in the emergency room, and I want to say that she is an ice cube. That is, I believe I can understand what's going on with her, that I can discern all her relevant properties. I believe I can help her.

Charlotte Duveen, as we will call her, is forty-nine years old, and for two days she has had abdominal pain. I begin observing her from the moment I walk through the curtains into her room. She is sitting cross-legged in the chair next to her stretcher and greets me with a cheerful, tobacco-beaten voice. She does not look sick. No clutching the belly. No gasping for words. Her color is good—neither flushed nor pale. Her shoulder-length brown hair has been brushed, her red lipstick neatly applied.

She tells me the pain started out crampy, like a gas pain. But then, during the course of the day, it became sharp and focused, and as she says this she points to a spot in the lower right part of her abdomen. She has developed diarrhea. She constantly feels as if she has to urinate. She doesn't have a fever. She is not nauseated. Actually, she is hungry. She tells me that she ate a hot dog at Fenway Park two days ago and visited the exotic birds at the zoo a few days before that, and she asks if either might have anything to do with this. She has two grown children. Her last period was three months ago. She smokes half a pack a day. She used to use heroin but says she's clean now. She once had hepatitis. She has never had surgery.

I feel her abdomen. It could be anything, I think: food poisoning, a virus, appendicitis, a urinary-tract infection, an ovarian cyst, a pregnancy. Her abdomen is soft, without distension, and there is an area of particular tenderness in the lower right quadrant. When I press there, I feel her muscles harden reflexively beneath my fingers. On the pelvic exam, her ovaries feel normal. I order some lab tests.

Her white blood cell count comes back elevated. Her urinalysis is normal. A pregnancy test is negative. I order an abdominal CT scan.

I am sure I can figure out what's wrong with her, but, if you think about it, that's a curious faith. I have never seen this woman before in my life, and yet I presume that she is like the others I've examined. Is it true? None of my other patients, admittedly, were forty-nine-year-old women who had had hepatitis and a drug habit, had recently been to the zoo and eaten a Fenway frank, and had come in with two days of mild lower-right-quadrant pain. Yet I still believe. Every day, we take people to surgery and open their abdomens, and, broadly speaking, we know what we will find: not eels or tiny chattering machines or a pool of blue liquid but coils of bowel, a liver to one side, a stomach to the other, a bladder down below. There are, of course, differences—an adhesion in one patient, an infection in another—but we have catalogued and sorted them by the thousands, making a statistical profile of mankind.

I am leaning toward appendicitis. The pain is in the right place. The timing of her symptoms, her exam, and her white blood cell count all fit with what I've seen before. She's hungry, however; she's walking around, not looking sick, and this seems unusual. I go to the radiology reading room and stand in the dark, looking over the radiologist's shoulder at the images of Duveen's abdomen flashing up on the monitor. He points to the appendix, wormlike, thick, surrounded by gray, streaky fat. It's appendicitis, he says confidently. I call the attending surgeon on duty and tell him what we've found. "Book the OR," he says. We're going to do an appendectomy.

This one is as sure as we get. Yet I've worked on similar cases in which we opened the patient up and found a normal appendix. Surgery itself is a kind of autopsy. "Autopsy" literally means "to see for oneself," and, despite our knowledge and technology, when we look we're often unprepared for what we find. Sometimes it turns out that we had missed a clue along the way, made a genuine mistake. Sometimes we turn out wrong despite doing everything right.

Whether with living patients or dead, however, we cannot know until we look. Even in the case of Mr. Sykes, I now wonder whether we put our stitches in correctly, or whether the bleeding had come from somewhere else entirely. Doctors are no longer asking such questions. Equally troubling, people seem happy to let us off the hook. In 1995, the United States National Center for Health Statistics stopped collecting autopsy statistics altogether. We can no longer even say how rare autopsies have become.

From what I've learned looking inside people, I've decided human beings are somewhere between a hurricane and an ice cube: in some respects, permanently mysterious, but in others—with enough science and careful probing—entirely scrutable. It would be as foolish to think we have reached the limits of human knowledge as it is to think we could ever know everything. There is still room enough to get better, to ask questions of even the dead, to learn from knowing when our simple certainties are wrong.

The Dead Baby Mystery

One by one, between 1949 and 1968, each of the ten children born to Marie Noe, a Philadelphia woman, died. One was stillborn. One died at the hospital just after birth. But eight others expired at home, just infants, in their cribs, where Noe said she found them blue and either limp or gasping. Doctors, including some of the most respected pathologists of the time, could find no explanation for the eight crib deaths—autopsies had in fact been done in every case. Foul play was strongly considered, but no evidence for it was found. Later, the medical community would come to recognize that thousands of seemingly healthy infants died inexplicably in their beds each year, a circumstance given the name Sudden Infant Death Syndrome, or SIDS, and the cases were attributed to this.

Still, eight unexplained baby deaths in one family do not sit easily. Marie Noe lost more babies than any mother ever known. We expect doctors to do better than the meager "Cause of death: Undetermined" that the pathologists put in the autopsy reports. Three decades later, they finally seemed to come through. On August 4, 1998, Philadelphia District Attorney Lynne Abraham cited new medical evidence to assert that Noe, now seventy, had smothered her children with a pillow. "Science," Abraham told the Associated Press, "has been solving old, unsolved cases." She charged Noe with eight counts of first degree murder.

Abraham's claim puzzled me. How did she—or rather, "science"—determine that the deaths were homicide and not SIDS? One of the great appeals of science is the idea that it can erase uncertainties. But the truth of the matter is that it tends to raise as many questions as it answers. And this situation seemed unlikely to be an exception. SIDS is not really a disease but rather the name doctors have given to one of the great medical mysteries of our time. Any sudden infant death that remains unexplained after a complete and inconclusive postmortem investigation is defined as SIDS. Typically in these cases, a previously healthy baby is found dead in bed. No cry is heard from the infant prior to its death. The child may be found with clenched fists or frothy, bloodstained fluid issuing from the nose and mouth. Although 90 percent of SIDS deaths occur by six months of age, older infants can die spontaneously and unexpectedly as well.

The early SIDS theory that the babies simply stop breathing has been discredited. Two suggestive findings are that sleeping on soft bedding and sleeping facedown both increase a baby's risk of sudden death. A successful campaign to get parents to put babies to bed on their backs or sides has been associated with a 38 percent drop in SIDS deaths over four years. Perhaps SIDS will turn out to be a kind of freak accident in which babies, unable to turn over, are smothered by their own bedding. The findings raise questions about how in the world you could accurately distinguish suffocation from SIDS—particularly in the Noe cases, in which the original autopsies had revealed no marks of force, and the corpses were now nothing but bone. Forensic pathologists and child abuse experts I contacted confirmed that there is no distinctive autopsy finding or new test that could distinguish SIDS from homicide by suffocation. So what was the actual basis for charging Noe?

Shortly after the charges were announced, I called around to various people involved in the case to ask that question. None would answer for attribution. But under promise of anonymity, an official admitted that there was no direct evidence to support the charges of homicide. In October 1997, after a reporter from *Philadelphia* magazine had begun making inquiries for an article about the Noe babies, Philadelphia homicide investigators decided to reopen the case. They asked the Philadelphia Medical Examiner's office to reexamine the previous autopsies—which really meant just reviewing the available autopsy reports (one was missing), death certificates, and investigation reports. The doctors found no missed physical signs of suffocation, no telltale, overlooked blood work or other tests. Just like the previous pathologists, all they had was eight infant deaths in one family without evidence of bodily harm and their suspicions about a mother who had been the only person present when each of the children died. The only difference was that this time the doctors were willing to declare that the pattern alone indicated that the manner of death was homicide.

In child abuse cases, as in so many things, science often can provide only circumstantial evidence. Occasionally, it is true, we doctors do find direct and convincing evidence for diagnosis: burns that could only be from cigarettes, bruises that trace the outline of a coat hanger, a uniform, stockinglike burn indicating a foot plunged into and held down in hot liquid. I once took care of a screaming two-month-old boy whose face had been badly scalded—his father said it was the result of accidentally turning on the hot water tap while bathing him. But the absence of a splash pattern to the burns made us on the team suspect abuse. We took full body X rays of the child to look for other injuries. He turned out to have between five and eight rib fractures and fractures of both legs. Some were weeks old. Some were new. Genetic and collagen studies excluded bone and metabolic abnormalities that could account for such extensive injuries. This was concrete evidence of abuse, and the child was removed from his parents. But even then, as my testimony at trial indicated, our evidence could not point to which of them had done the harm. (It was the police investigation that ultimately clinched the case against the father and led a jury to send him to jail for felony child abuse.) Most cases do not come with such obvious physical signs of maltreatment. In deciding whether to sic the department of social services or police on a family, we usually have only vague indicators to rely upon. According to guidelines used at Children's Hospital in Boston, for example, *any* bruise, facial laceration, or long-bone fracture in an infant is supposed to be considered evidence of possible abuse. That's not much to go on. In the end, doctors look for the parents to tell us much more than any physical evidence can.

A few years ago, my one-year-old daughter Hattie was playing in our playroom when suddenly she let out a blood-curdling scream. My wife ran in and found her lying on the ground, her right arm bent midway between the elbow and the wrist like an extra joint. As near as we could figure, it seemed she had tried to climb onto our futon couch, gotten her arm caught in the slats, and then gotten pushed over inadvertently by Walker, then two years old. As she fell, the bones of her forearm broke in two. When I arrived with her at the hospital, I was grilled by three different people asking me over and over again, "Now, exactly how did this happen?" It was, I knew all too well, a suspicious story—an unwitnessed fall resulting in a bad long-bone fracture. The doctors were looking, as I do with any child trauma victim, for any inconsistencies or changes in the story the parents tell. It is easy for parents to feel angry and self-righteous when doctors ask questions as if they are cops, but as advanced as medicine has become, questions are still our main diagnostic test for the presence of abuse.

Ultimately, I must have allayed any concerns. My daughter got a pink cast, and I took her home without incident. I couldn't help but think, however, that my social status played a role in all this. As much as doctors may try to avoid it, when we decide whether to call officials in a case, social factors inevitably play a role. We know, for example, that single parents have almost double the risk of being abusive, poor families almost sixteen times the likelihood. We know that one-third of crack-using mothers abuse or neglect their children. (Race, by the way, is not a factor.) The profile is always in mind.

In the case of Marie Noe, the factors likewise played to her advantage. She was married, middle-class, and respectable. But the fact of eight deaths must mean something, right? As one medical examiner involved in the reopened cases said, repeating a maxim that has gained currency among pathologists, "One SIDS death is a tragedy. Two is a mystery. Three is murder."

The real answer, however, is that while the pattern seems damning enough in itself, it cannot satisfy reasonable doubts. Bucking his colleagues, Pittsburgh Medical Examiner Cyril Wecht asserted flatly that multiple SIDS deaths in one family do not automatically mean murder. The numbers certainly make the Noe deaths suspicious, he said. After all, experts now believe that losing one baby to SIDS does not increase the chances that a family will lose another. Having even two deaths in one family certainly merits investigation. But, as Wecht went on, there have been cases of two and three unexplained infant deaths in a family in which homicide was ruled highly unlikely. Parents of SIDS babies have been wrongly accused in the past. And most troubling, we don't know what SIDS is in the first place. We may have lumped several different diseases together in describing the syndrome. Perhaps multiple natural deaths in a family will prove possible, though undoubtedly rare.

Still, although science often cannot prove even fatal child abuse, science is not without its power. Confronted during police questioning with the medical "proof" of her homicides, Noe admitted to having suffocated four of her children and said that she couldn't recall what had happened to the others. Her lawyer immediately challenged the reliability and admissibility of the confession, obtained as it was during an all-night interview. On June 28, 1999, however,

Marie Noe stood up in a Philadelphia Common Pleas Court room, steadied herself with her cane, and pleaded guilty to eight counts of second-degree murder. Sitting in the gallery, her seventy-seven-year-old husband, Arthur, shook his head in bewilderment.

In the end, it is sometimes not science but what people tell us that is the most convincing proof we have.

Whose Body Is It, Anyway?

The first time I saw the patient it was the day before his surgery, and I thought he might be dead. Joseph Lazaroff, as I'll call him, lay in bed, his eyes closed, a sheet pulled up over his thin, birdlike chest. When people are asleep—or even when they are anesthetized and not breathing by themselves—it does not occur to you to question whether they are alive. They exude life as if it were heat. It's visible in the tone of an arm muscle, the supple curve of their lips, the flush of their skin. But as I bent forward to tap Lazaroff on the shoulder I found myself stopping short with that instinctive apprehension of touching the dead. His color was all wrong—pallid, fading. His cheeks, eyes, and temples were sunken, and his skin was stretched over his face like a mask. Strangest of all, his head was suspended two inches above his pillow, as if rigor mortis had set in.

"Mr. Lazaroff?" I called out, and his eyes opened. He looked at me without interest, silent and motionless.

I was in my first year of surgical residency and was working on the neurosurgery team at the time. Lazaroff had a cancer that had spread throughout his body, and he had been scheduled for surgery to excise a tumor from his spine. The senior resident had sent me to "consent" him—that is, to get Lazaroff's signature giving final permission for the operation. No problem, I had said. But now, looking at this frail, withered man, I had to wonder if we were right to operate on him.

His patient chart told the story. Eight months earlier, he had seen his doctor about a backache. The doctor initially found nothing suspicious, but three months later the pain had worsened and he ordered a scan. It revealed extensive cancer—multiple tumors in Lazaroff's liver, bowel, and up and down his spine. A biopsy revealed it was an untreatable cancer.

Lazaroff was only in his early sixties, a longtime city administrator who had a touch of diabetes, the occasional angina, and the hardened manner of a man who had lost his wife a few years earlier and learned to live alone. His condition deteriorated rapidly. In a matter of months, he lost more than fifty pounds. As the tumors in his abdomen grew, his belly, scrotum, and legs filled up with fluid. The pain and debility eventually made it impossible for him to keep working. His thirty-something son moved in to care for him. Lazaroff went on around-the-clock morphine to control his pain. His doctors told him that he might have only weeks to live. Lazaroff wasn't ready to hear it, though. He still talked about the day he'd go back to work.

Then he took several bad falls; his legs had become unaccountably weak. He also became incontinent. He went back to his oncologist. A scan showed that a metastasis was compressing his thoracic spinal cord. The oncologist admitted him to the hospital and tried a round of radiation, but it had no effect. Indeed, he became unable to move his right leg; his lower body was becoming paralyzed.

He had two options left. He could undergo spinal surgery. It wouldn't cure him—surgery or not, he had at the most a few months left—but it offered a last-ditch chance of halting the progression of spinal-cord damage and possibly restoring some strength to his legs and sphincters. The risks, however, were severe. We'd have to go in through his chest and collapse his lung just to get at his spine. He'd face a long, difficult, and painful recovery. And given his frail condition—not to mention the previous history of heart disease—his chances of surviving the procedure and getting back home were slim.

The alternative was to do nothing. He'd go home and continue with hospice care, which would keep him comfortable and help him maintain a measure of control over his life. The immobility and incontinence would certainly worsen. But it was his best chance of dying peacefully, in his own bed, and being able to say good-bye to his loved ones.

The decision was Lazaroff's.

That, in itself, is a remarkable fact. Little more than a decade ago, doctors made the decisions; patients did what they were told. Doctors did not consult patients about their desires and priorities, and routinely withheld information—sometimes crucial information, such as what drugs they were on, what treatments they were being given, and what their diagnosis was. Patients were even forbidden to look at their own medical records: it wasn't their property, doctors said. They were regarded as children: too fragile and simpleminded to handle the truth, let alone make decisions. And they suffered for it. People were put on machines, given drugs, and subjected to operations they would not have chosen. And they missed out on treatments that they might have preferred.

My father recounts that, through the 1970s and much of the 1980s, when men came to see him seeking vasectomies, it was accepted that he would judge whether the surgery was not only medically appropriate but also personally appropriate for them. He routinely refused to do the operation if the men were unmarried, married but without children, or "too young." In retrospect, he's not sure he did right by all these patients, and, he says, he'd never do things this way today. In fact, he can't even think of a patient in the last few years whom he has turned down for a vasectomy.

One of the reasons for this dramatic shift in how decisions are made in medicine was a 1984 book, *The Silent World of Doctor and Patient*, by a Yale doctor and ethicist named Jay Katz. It was a devastating critique of traditional medical decision making, and it had wide influence. In the book, Katz argued that medical decisions could and should be made by the patients involved. And he made his case using the stories of actual patients.

One was that of "Iphigenia Jones," a twenty-one-year-old woman who was found to have a malignancy in one of her breasts. Then, as now, she had two options: mastectomy (which would mean removing the breast and the lymph nodes of the nearby axilla) or radiation with minimal surgery (removing just the lump and the lymph nodes). Survival rates were equal, although in a spared breast the tumor can recur and ultimately make mastectomy necessary. This surgeon preferred doing mastectomies, and that's what he told her he'd do. In the days leading up to the operation, however, the surgeon developed misgivings about removing the breast of someone that young. So the night before the operation he did an unusual thing: he discussed the treatment options with her and let her choose. She chose the breast-preserving treatment.

Sometime later, both patient and surgeon appeared on a panel discussing treatment options for breast cancer. Their story drew a heated response. Surgeons almost uniformly attacked the idea that patients should be allowed to choose. As one surgeon asked, "If doctors have such trouble deciding which treatment is best, how can patients decide?" But, as Katz wrote, the decision involved not technical but personal issues: Which was more important to Iphigenia—the preservation of her breast or the security of living without a significant chance that the lump would grow back? No doctor was the authority on these matters. Only Iphigenia was. Yet in such situations doctors did step in, often not even asking about a patient's concerns, and made their own decisions—decisions perhaps influenced by money, professional bias (for example, surgeons tend to favor surgery), and personal idiosyncrasy.

Eventually, medical schools came around to Katz's position. By the time I attended, in the early 1990s, we were taught to see patients as autonomous decision makers. "You work for them," I was often reminded. There are still many old-school doctors who try to dictate from on high, but they are finding that patients won't put up with that anymore. Most doctors, taking seriously the idea that patients should control their own fates, lay out the options and the risks involved. A few even refuse to make recommendations, for fear of improperly influencing patients. Patients ask questions, look up information on the Internet, seek second opinions. And they decide.

In practice, however, matters aren't so straightforward. Patients, it turns out, make bad decisions, too. Sometimes, of course, the difference between one option and another isn't especially significant. But when you see your patient making a grave mistake, should you simply do what the patient wants? The current medical orthodoxy says yes. After all, whose body is it, anyway?

Lazaroff wanted surgery. The oncologist was dubious about the choice, but she called in a neurosurgeon. The neurosurgeon, a trim man in his forties with a stellar reputation and a fondness for bow ties, saw Lazaroff and his son that afternoon. He warned them at length about how terrible the risks were and how limited the potential benefit. Sometimes, he told me later, patients just don't seem to hear the dangers, and in those cases he tends to be especially explicit about them—getting stuck on a ventilator because of poor lung function, having a stroke, dying. But Lazaroff wasn't to be dissuaded. The surgeon put him on the schedule.

"Mr. Lazaroff, I'm a surgical resident, and I'm here to talk to you about your surgery tomorrow," I said. "You're going to be having a thoracic spine corpectomy and fusion." He looked at me blankly. "This means that we will be removing the tumor compressing your spine," I said. His expression did not change. "The hope is that it will keep your paralysis from worsening."

"I'm not paralyzed," he said at last. "The surgery is so I won't become paralyzed."

I quickly retreated. "I'm sorry—I meant, keep you from becoming paralyzed." Perhaps this was just semantics—he could still move his left leg some. "I just need you to sign a permission form so you can have the surgery tomorrow."

The "informed-consent form" is a relatively recent development. It lists as many complications as we doctors can think of—everything from a mild allergic reaction to death—and, in signing it, you indicate that you have accepted these risks. It has the mark of lawyerdom and bureaucracy, and I doubt that patients feel any better informed after reading it. It does, however, provide an occasion to review the risks involved.

The neurosurgeon had already gone over them in detail. So I hit the highlights. "We ask for your signature so we're sure you understand the risks," I said. "Although you're having this done to preserve your abilities, the operation could fail or leave you paralyzed." I tried to sound firm without being harsh. "You could have a stroke or a heart attack or could even die." I held the form and a pen out to him.

"No one said I could die from this," he said, tremulously. "It's my last hope. Are you saying I'm going to die?"

I froze, not knowing quite what to say. Just then, Lazaroff's son, whom I'll call David, arrived, with his wrinkled clothes, scraggly beard, and slight paunch. The father's mood changed abruptly, and I remembered from notes in the medical chart that David had recently raised the question with him of whether heroic measures were still appropriate. "Don't you give up on me," Lazaroff now rasped at his son. "You give me every chance I've got." He snatched the form and the pen from my hand. We stood, chastised and silent, as Lazaroff made a slow, illegible scrawl near the line for his signature.

Outside the room, David told me that he wasn't sure this was the right move. His mother had spent a long time in intensive care on a ventilator before dying of emphysema, and since then his father had often said that he did not want anything like that to happen to him. But now he was adamant about doing "everything." David did not dare argue with him.

Lazaroff had his surgery the next day. Once under anesthesia, he was rolled onto his left side. A thoracic surgeon made a long incision, opening into the chest cavity from the front around to the back along the eighth rib, slipped in a rib spreader, cranked it open, and then fixed in place a retractor to hold the deflated lung out of the way. You could see right down into the back of the chest to the spinal column. A fleshy, tennis ball–size mass enveloped the tenth vertebra. The neurosurgeon took over and meticulously dissected around and under the tumor. It took a couple of hours, but eventually the tumor was attached only where it invaded the bony vertebral body. He then used a rongeur—a rigid, jawed instrument—to take small, painstaking bites in the vertebral body, like a beaver gnawing slowly through a tree trunk, ultimately removing the vertebra and, with it, the mass. To rebuild the spine, he filled the space left behind with a doughy plug of methacrylate, an acrylic cement, and let it slowly harden in place. He slipped a probe in behind the new artificial vertebra. There was plenty of space. It had taken more than four hours, but the pressure on the spinal cord was gone. The thoracic surgeon closed Lazaroff's chest, leaving a rubber chest tube jutting out to reinflate his lung, and he was wheeled into intensive care.

The operation was a technical success. Lazaroff's lungs wouldn't recover, however, and we struggled to get him off the ventilator. Over the next few days, they gradually became stiff and fibrotic, requiring higher ventilator pressures. We tried to keep him under sedation, but he frequently broke through and woke up wild-eyed and thrashing. David kept a despondent bedside vigil. Successive chest X rays showed worsening lung damage. Small blood clots lodged in Lazaroff's lungs, and we put him on a blood thinner to prevent more clots from forming. Then some slow bleeding started—we weren't sure from where—and we had to give him blood transfusions almost daily. After a week, he began spiking fevers, but we couldn't find where the infection was. On the ninth day after the operation, the high ventilator pressures blew small holes in his lungs. We had to cut into his chest and insert an extra tube to keep his lungs from collapsing. The effort and expense it took to keep him going were enormous, the results dispiriting. It became apparent that our efforts were futile. It was exactly the way Lazaroff hadn't wanted to die—strapped down and sedated, tubes in every natural orifice and in several new ones, and on a ventilator. On the fourteenth day, David told the neurosurgeon that we should stop.

The neurosurgeon came to me with the news. I went to Lazaroff's ICU room, one of eight bays arrayed in a semicircle around a nursing station, each with a tile floor, a window, and a sliding glass door that closed it off from the noise but not from the eyes of the nurses. A nurse and I slipped in. I checked to make sure that Lazaroff's morphine drip was turned up high. Taking my place at the bedside, I leaned close to him and, in case he could hear me, told him I was going to take the breathing tube out of his mouth. I snipped the ties securing the tube and deflated the balloon cuff holding it in his trachea. Then I pulled the tube out. He coughed a couple of times, opened his eyes briefly, and then closed them. The nurse suctioned out phlegm from his mouth. I turned the ventilator off, and suddenly the room was quiet except for the sound of his labored, gasping breaths. We watched as he tired out. His breathing slowed down until he took only occasional, agonal breaths, and then he stopped. I put my stethoscope on his chest and listened to his heart fade away. Thirteen minutes after I took him off the ventilator, I told the nurse to record that Joseph Lazaroff had died.

Lazaroff, I thought, chose badly. Not, however, because he died so violently and appallingly. Good decisions can have bad results (sometimes people must take terrible chances), and bad decisions can have good results ("Better lucky than good," surgeons like to say). I thought Lazaroff chose badly because his choice ran against his deepest interests—interests not as I or anyone else conceived them, but as he conceived them. Above all, it was clear that he wanted to live. He would take any risk—even death—to live. But, as we explained to him, life was not what we had to offer. We could offer only a chance of preserving minimal lower-body function for his brief remaining time—at a cost of severe violence to him and against extreme odds of a miserable death. But he did not hear us: in staving off paralysis, he seemed to believe that he might stave off death. There are people who will look clear-eyed at such odds and take their chances with surgery. But, knowing how much Lazaroff had dreaded dying the way his wife had, I do not believe he was one of them.

Could it have been a mistake, then, even to have told him about the surgical option? Our contemporary medical credo has made us exquisitely attuned to the requirements of patient autonomy. But there are still times—and they are more frequent than we readily admit—when a doctor has to steer patients to do what's right for themselves.

This is a controversial suggestion. People are rightly suspicious of those claiming to know better than they do what's best for them. But a good physician cannot simply stand aside when patients make bad or self-defeating decisions—decisions that go against their deepest goals.

I remember a case from my first weeks of internship. I was on the general surgical service, and among the patients I was responsible for was a woman in her fifties—I'll call her Mrs. McLaughlin—who had had a big abdominal operation just two days before. An incision ran the entire length of her belly. Fluids and pain medication dripped through an intravenous line into her arm. She was recovering according to schedule, but she wouldn't get out of bed. I explained why it was essential for her to get up and around: it cuts the risk of pneumonia, clot formation in leg veins, and other detrimental effects. She wasn't swayed. She was tired, she said, and didn't feel up to it. Did she understand that she was risking serious problems? Yes, she said. Just leave me be.

During rounds that afternoon, the chief resident asked me if the patient had gotten out of bed. Well, no, I said—she had refused. That's no excuse, the chief said, and she marched me back to Mrs. McLaughlin's room. The chief sat down on the edge of the bed and, as friendly as a country pastor, said, "Hi, how're you doing," made some small talk, took Mrs. McLaughlin by the hand, and then said, "It's time to get out of bed now." And I watched Mrs. McLaughlin get up without a moment's hesitation, shuffle over to a chair, plop herself down, and say, "You know, that wasn't so bad after all."

I had come into residency to learn how to be a surgeon. I had thought that meant simply learning the repertoire of moves and techniques involved in doing an operation or making a diagnosis. In fact, there was also the new and delicate matter of talking patients through their decisions—something that sometimes entailed its own repertoire of moves and techniques.

Suppose you're a doctor. You're in an examination room of your clinic—one of those cramped spaces with fluorescent lights, a Matisse poster on the wall, a box of latex gloves on the counter, and a cold, padded patient table as centerpiece—seeing a female patient in her forties. She's a mother of two and a partner in a downtown law firm. Despite the circumstances, and the flimsy paper gown she's in, she manages to maintain her composure. You feel no mass or abnormality in her breasts. She had a mammogram before seeing you, and now you review the radiologist's report, which reads, "There is a faint group of punctate, clustered calcifications in the upper outer quadrant of the left breast that were not clearly present on the prior examination. Biopsy must be considered to exclude the possibility of malignancy." Translation: worrisome features have appeared; they could mean breast cancer.

You tell her the news. Given the findings, you say, you think she ought to have a biopsy. She groans, and then stiffens. "Every time I see one of you people, you find something you want biopsied," she says. Three times in the past five years, her annual mammogram has revealed an area of "suspicious" calcifications. Three times a surgeon has taken her to the operating room and removed the tissue in question. And three times, under the pathologist's microscope, it has proved to be benign. "You just don't know when enough is enough," she says. "Whatever these specks are that keep turning up, they've proved to be normal." She pauses, and decides. "I'm not getting another goddam biopsy," she says, and she stands up to get dressed.

Do you let her go? It's not an unreasonable thing to do. She's an adult, after all. And a biopsy is not a small thing. Scattered across her left breast are the raised scars—one almost three inches long. Enough tissue has already been taken out that the left breast is distinctly smaller than the right one. And, yes, there are doctors who biopsy too much, who take out breast tissue on the most equivocal of findings. Patients are often right to push for explanations and second opinions.

Still, these calcifications are not equivocal findings. They commonly do indicate cancer—even if they don't always—and typically at an early and treatable stage. Now, if having control over one's life is to mean anything, people have to be permitted to make their own mistakes. But when the stakes are this high, and a bad choice may be irreversible, doctors are reluctant to sit back. This is when they tend to push.

So push. Your patient is getting ready to walk out the door. You could stop her in her tracks and tell her she's making a big mistake. Give her a heavy speech about cancer. Point out the fallacy in supposing that three negative biopsies proves that the fourth one will be negative as well. And in all likelihood you'll lose her. The aim isn't to show her how wrong she is. The aim is to give her the chance to change her own mind.

Here's what I've seen good doctors do. They don't jump right in. They step out for a minute and give the woman time to get dressed. They take her down to the office to sit and talk, where it's more congenial and less antiseptic—with comfortable chairs instead of a hard table, a throw rug instead of linoleum. And, often, they don't stand or assume the throne behind the big oak desk but pull up a chair and sit with her. As one surgical professor told me, when you sit close by, on the same level as your patients, you're no longer the rushed, bossy doctor with no time to talk; patients feel less imposed upon and more inclined to consider that you may both be on the same side of the issue at hand.

Even at this point, many doctors won't fuss or debate. Instead, some have what can seem like strange, almost formulaic conversations with the patient, repeating, virtually word for word, what she tells them. "I see your point," they might say. "Every time you come in, we find something to biopsy. The specks keep coming up normal, but we never stop biopsying." Beyond this, many doctors say almost nothing until they're asked to. Whether one calls this a ruse or just being open to their patients, it works, oddly enough, nine times out of ten. People feel heard and like they have had an opportunity to express their beliefs and concerns. At that point, they may finally begin to ask questions, voice doubts, even work through the logic themselves. And once they do, they tend to come around.

A few still resist, though, and when doctors really think someone is endangering himself or herself, other tactics are not beyond the pale. They may enlist reinforcements. "Should we call the radiologist and see what he really thinks?" they might ask, or "Your family's out in the waiting room. Why don't we ask them to come in?" They might give the patient time "to think it over," knowing that people often waver and change their minds. Sometimes they resort to subtler dynamics. I once saw a doctor, faced with a heart disease patient who wouldn't consider quitting smoking, simply fall silent, letting the complete extent of his disappointment show. The seconds tocked by until a full minute had passed. Before a thoughtful, concerned, and, yes, sometimes crafty doctor, few patients will not eventually "choose" what the doctor recommends.

But it's misleading to view all this simply as the art of doctorly manipulation: when you see patients cede authority to the doctor, something else may be going on. The new orthodoxy about patient autonomy has a hard time acknowledging an awkward truth: patients frequently don't want the freedom that we've given them. That is, they're glad to have their autonomy respected, but the exercise of that autonomy means being able to relinquish it. Thus, it turns out that patients commonly prefer to have others make their medical decisions. One study found that although 64 percent of the general public thought they'd want to select their own treatment if they developed cancer, only 12 percent of newly diagnosed cancer patients actually did want to do so.

This dynamic is something I only came to understand recently. My youngest child, Hunter, was born five weeks early, weighing barely four pounds, and when she was eleven days old she stopped breathing. She had been home a week and doing well. That morning, however, she seemed irritable and fussy, and her nose ran. Thirty minutes after her feeding, her respiration became rapid, and she began making little grunting noises with each breath. Suddenly, Hunter stopped breathing. My wife, panicked, leaped up and shook Hunter awake, and the baby started breathing again. We rushed her to the hospital.

Fifteen minutes later, we were in a large, bright, emergency department examination room. With an oxygen mask on, Hunter didn't quite stabilize—she was still taking over sixty breaths a minute and expending all her energy to do it—but she regained normal oxygen levels in her blood and held her own. The doctors weren't sure what the cause of her trouble was. It could have been a heart defect, a bacterial infection, a virus. They took X rays, blood, and urine, did an electrocardiogram, and tapped her spinal fluid. They suspected—correctly, as it turned out—that the problem was an ordinary respiratory virus that her lungs were too little and immature to handle. But the results from the cultures wouldn't be back for a couple of days. They admitted her to the intensive care unit. That night, she began to tire out. She had several spells of apnea—periods of up to sixty seconds in which she stopped breathing, her heartbeat slowed, and she became pale and ominously still—but each time she came back, all by herself.

A decision needed to be made. Should she be intubated and put on a ventilator? Or should the doctors wait to see if she could recover without it? There were risks either way. If the team didn't intubate her now, under controlled circumstances, and she "crashed"—maybe the next time she would not wake up from an apneic spell—they would have to perform an emergency intubation, a tricky thing to do in a child so small. Delays could occur, the breathing tube could go down the wrong pipe, the doctors could inadvertently traumatize the airway and cause it to shut down, and then she might suffer brain damage or even die from lack of oxygen. The likelihood of such a disaster was slim but real. I myself had seen it happen. On the other hand, you don't want to put someone on a ventilator if you don't have to, least of all a small child. Serious and detrimental effects, such as pneumonia or the sort of lung blowout that Lazaroff experienced, happen frequently. And, as people who have been hooked up to one of these contraptions will tell you, the machine shoots air into and out of you with terrifying, uncomfortable force; your mouth becomes sore; your lips crack. Sedation is given, but the drugs bring complications, too.

So who should have made the choice? In many ways, I was the ideal candidate to decide what was best. I was the father, so I cared more than any hospital staffer ever could about which risks were taken. And I was a doctor, so I understood the issues involved. I also knew how often problems like miscommunication, overwork, and plain hubris could lead physicians to make bad choices.

And yet when the team of doctors came to talk to me about whether to intubate Hunter, I wanted them to decide—doctors I had never met before. The ethicist Jay Katz and others have disparaged this kind of desire as "childlike regression." But that judgment seems heartless to me. The uncertainties were savage, and I could not bear the possibility of making the wrong call. Even if I made what I was sure was the right choice for her, I could not live with the guilt if something went wrong. Some believe that patients should be pushed to take responsibility for decisions. But that would have seemed equally like a kind of harsh paternalism in itself. I needed Hunter's physicians to bear the responsibility: they could live with the consequences, good or bad.

I let the doctors make the call, and they did so on the spot. They would keep Hunter off the ventilator, they told me. And, with that, the bleary-eyed, stethoscope-collared pack shuffled onward to their next patient. Still, there was the nagging question: if I wanted the best decision for Hunter, was relinquishing my hard-won autonomy really the right thing to do? Carl Schneider, a professor of law and medicine at the University of Michigan, recently published a book called *The Practice of Autonomy*, in which he sorted through a welter of studies and data on medical decision making, even undertaking a systematic analysis of patients' memoirs. He found that the ill were often in a poor position to make good choices: they were frequently exhausted, irritable, shattered, or despondent. Often, they were just trying to get through their immediate pain, nausea, and fatigue; they could hardly think about major decisions. This rang true to me. I wasn't even the patient, and all I could do was sit and watch Hunter, worry, or distract myself with busywork. I did not have the concentration or the energy to weigh the treatment options properly.

Schneider found that physicians, being less emotionally engaged, are able to reason through the uncertainties without the distortions of fear and attachment. They work in a scientific culture that disciplines the way they make decisions. They have the benefit of "group rationality"—norms based on scholarly literature and refined practice. And they have the key relevant experience. Even though I am a doctor, I did not have the experience that Hunter's doctors had with her specific condition.

In the end, Hunter managed to stay off the ventilator, although she had a slow and sometimes scary recovery. At one point, less than twenty-four hours after the doctors had transferred her to a regular floor, her condition deteriorated and they had to rush her back to the

ICU. She spent ten days in intensive care and two weeks in the hospital. But she went home in fine shape.

Just as there is an art to being a doctor, there is an art to being a patient. You must choose wisely when to submit and when to assert yourself. Even when patients decide not to decide, they should still question their physicians and insist on explanations. I may have let Hunter's doctors take control, but I pressed them for a clear plan in the event that she should crash. Later, I worried that they were being too slow to feed her—she wasn't given anything to eat for more than a week, and I pestered them with questions as to why. When they took her off the oxygen monitor on her eleventh day in the hospital, I got nervous. What harm was there in keeping it on, I asked. I'm sure I was obstinate, even wrongheaded, at times. You do the best you can, taking the measure of your doctors and nurses and your own situation, trying to be neither too passive nor too pushy for your own good.

But the conundrum remains: if both doctors and patients are fallible, who should decide? We want a rule. And so we've decided that patients should be the ultimate arbiter. But such a hard-and-fast rule seems ill-suited both to a caring relationship between doctor and patient and to the reality of medical care, where a hundred decisions have to be made quickly. A mother is in labor: should the doctor give hormones to stimulate stronger contractions? Should he or she break the bag of water? Should an epidural anesthetic be given? If so, at what point in labor? Are antibiotics needed? How often should the mother's blood pressure be checked? Should the doctor use forceps? Should the doctor perform an episiotomy? If things don't progress quickly, should the doctor perform a cesarean section? The doctor should not make all these decisions, and neither should the patient. Something must be worked out between them, one on one—a personal modus operandi.

Where many ethicists go wrong is in promoting patient autonomy as a kind of ultimate value in medicine rather than recognizing it as one value among others. Schneider found that what patients want most from doctors isn't autonomy per se; it's competence and kindness. Now, kindness will often involve respecting patients' autonomy, assuring that they have control over vital decisions. But it may also mean taking on burdensome decisions when patients don't want to make them, or guiding patients in the right direction when they do. Even when patients do want to make their own decisions, there are times when the compassionate thing to do is to press hard: to steer them to accept an operation or treatment that they fear, or forgo one that they'd pinned their hopes on. Many ethicists find this line of reasoning disturbing, and medicine will continue to struggle with how patients and doctors ought to make decisions. But, as the field grows ever more complex and technological, the real task isn't to banish paternalism; the real task is to preserve kindness.

One more case, again from my internship year. The patient—I'll call him Mr. Howe—was in his late thirties, stout, bald, and with a muted, awkward manner. I wanted to turn the sound up when he spoke, and pictured him as someone who worked alone, perhaps as an accountant or a computer programmer. He was in the hospital following an operation for a badly infected gallbladder. Whenever I saw him, he wore the sad look of someone caged, and he asked no questions. He could not wait to leave the hospital.

Late Saturday afternoon, maybe three days after his surgery, his nurse paged me. He had spiked a high fever and become short of breath. He didn't look well, she said.

I found him sweating profusely, his face flushed, eyes wide. He was sitting bent forward, propped up on his thick arms, panting. He had an oxygen mask on, and, even with the flow turned up to the maximum, the pulse-oximeter readings showed barely adequate oxygen levels in his blood. His heart was racing at well over a hundred beats a minute, and his blood pressure was much too low.

His wife, a small, thin, pale woman with lank black hair, stood to the side, rocking on her feet and hugging herself. I examined

Mr. Howe, drew blood for tests and cultures, and asked the nurse to give him a bolus of intravenous fluid, trying to appear as confident as I could. Then I went out into the hall and paged K., one of the chief residents, for help.

When she called back, I filled her in on the details. I think he's septic, I said. Sometimes a bacterial infection gets into the bloodstream and triggers a massive, system-wide response: high fevers and dilation of the body's peripheral blood vessels, causing the skin to flush, the blood pressure to drop, and the heart to speed up. After abdominal surgery, a common cause of this is an infection of the surgical wound. But his incision was not red or hot or tender, and he had no pain in his belly. His lungs, however, had sounded like a washing machine when I listened with my stethoscope. Perhaps a pneumonia had started this disaster.

K. came right over. She was just past thirty, almost six feet tall, with short blond hair, athletic, exhaustingly energetic, and relentlessly can-do. She took one look at Howe and then murmured to the nurse to keep an intubation kit available at the bedside. I had started antibiotics, and the fluids had improved his blood pressure a bit, but he was still on maximal oxygen and working hard to maintain his breathing. She went over to him, put a hand on his shoulder, and asked how he was doing. It took a moment before he managed to reply. "Fine," he said—a silly answer to a silly question, but a conversation starter. She explained the situation: the sepsis, the likely pneumonia, and the probability that he would get worse before he got better. The antibiotics would fix the problem, but not instantly, she said, and he was tiring out quickly. To get him through it, she would need to put him to sleep, intubate him, and place him on a breathing machine.

"No," he gasped, and sat straight up. "Don't . . . put me . . . on a . . . machine."

It would not be for long, she said. Maybe a couple of days. We'd give him sedatives so he'd be as comfortable as possible the whole time. And—she wanted to be sure he understood—without the ventilator he would die.

He shook his head. "No . . . machine!"

He was, we believed, making a bad decision — out of fear, maybe incomprehension. With antibiotics and some high-tech support, we had every reason to believe, he'd recover fully. Howe had a lot to live for — he was young and otherwise healthy, and he had a wife and a child. Apparently, he thought so, too, for he had cared enough about his well-being to accept the initial operation. If not for the terror of the moment, we thought, he would have accepted the treatment. Could we be certain we were right? No, but if we were right could we really just let him die?

K. looked over at Howe's wife, who was stricken with fear and, in an effort to enlist her in the cause, asked what she thought her husband should do. She burst into tears. "I don't know, I don't know," she cried. "Can't you save him?" She couldn't take it anymore, and left the room. For the next few minutes, K. kept trying to persuade Howe. When it was clear that she was making no headway, she left to phone his attending surgeon at home, and then returned to the bedside. Soon Howe did tire out. He leaned back in his bed, pale, sweaty strands of hair sticking to his pate, oxygen levels dropping on the monitor. He closed his eyes, and he gradually fell into unconsciousness.

That was when K. went into action. She lowered the head of Howe's bed until he lay flat. She had a nurse draw up a tranquilizing agent and administer it in his IV. She pressed a bag mask to his face and squeezed breaths of oxygen down into his lungs. Then I handed her the intubation equipment, and she slipped a long, clear plastic breathing tube down into his trachea on the first try. We wheeled Howe in his bed to the elevator and took him down a few floors to the intensive care unit.

Later, I found his wife and explained that he was now on a ventilator in the ICU. She said nothing and went to see him.

Over the next twenty-four hours, his lungs improved markedly. We lightened up on the sedation and let him take over breathing from the machine. He woke up and opened his eyes, the breathing tube sticking out of his mouth. He did not struggle.

"I'm going to take this tube out of your mouth now, OK?" I said. He nodded. I cut the ties and deflated the balloon cuff holding the tube in place. Then I pulled it out, and he coughed violently a few times. "You had pneumonia," I told him, "but you're doing just fine now."

I stood there silent and anxious for a moment, waiting to see what he would say. He swallowed hard, wincing from the soreness. Then he looked at me, and, in a hoarse but steady voice, he said, "Thank you."

The Case of the Red Leg

Seeing patients with one of the surgery professors in his clinic one afternoon, I was struck by how often he had to answer his patients' questions, "I do not know." These are four little words a doctor tends to be reluctant to utter. We're supposed to have the answers. We want to have the answers. But there was not a single person he did not have to say those four little words to that day.

There was the patient who had come in two weeks after an abdominal hernia repair: "What's this pain I feel next to the wound?"

There was the patient one month after a gastric-bypass operation: "Why haven't I lost weight yet?"

There was the patient with a large pancreatic cancer: "Can you get it out?"

And to all, the attending gave the same reply: "I do not know."

A doctor still must have a plan, though. So to the hernia patient, he said, "Come back in a week and let's see how the pain's doing." To the gastric-bypass patient, "It'll be all right," and asked her to come back in a month. To the cancer patient, "We can try to get it out" — and although another surgeon thought he shouldn't (given the tumor's appearance on a scan, operation would be futile and risky, the colleague said), and he himself thought the odds of success were slim at best, he and the patient (who was only in her forties, with still-young children at home) decided to go ahead.

The core predicament of medicine—the thing that makes being a patient so wrenching, being a doctor so difficult, and being a part of a society that pays the bills they run up so vexing—is uncertainty. With all that we know nowadays about people and diseases and how to diagnose and treat them, it can be hard to see this, hard to grasp how deeply the uncertainty runs. As a doctor, you come to find, however, that the struggle in caring for people is more often with what you do not know than what you do. Medicine's ground state is uncertainty. And wisdom—for both patients and doctors—is defined by how one copes with it.

This is the story of one decision under uncertainty.

It was two o'clock on a Tuesday afternoon in June. I was in the middle of a seven-week stint as the senior surgical resident in the emergency room. I had just finished admitting someone with a gallbladder infection and was attempting to sneak out for a bite to eat when one of the emergency room physicians stopped me with yet another patient to see: a twenty-three-year-old, Eleanor Bratton, with a red and swollen leg. (The names of patients and colleagues have been changed.) "It's probably only a cellulitis"—a simple skin infection—"but it's a bad one," he said. He had started her on some intravenous antibiotics and admitted her to the medical service. But he wanted me to make sure there wasn't anything "surgical" going on—an abscess that needed draining or some such. "Would you mind taking a quick look?" Groan. No. Of course not.

She was in the observation unit, a separate, quieter ward within the ER where she could get antibiotics pumped into her arm and wait for admitting to find her a bed upstairs. The unit's nine beds are arrayed in a semicircle, each separated by a thin blue curtain, and I found her in Bed 1. She looked fit, athletic, and almost teenage, with blond hair tight in a ponytail, nails painted gold, and her eyes fixed on a television. There did not seem anything seriously ill about her.

She was lying comfortably, a sheet pulled up to her waist, the head of the bed raised. I glanced at her chart and saw that she had good vital signs, no fever, and no past medical problems. I walked up and introduced myself: "Hi, I'm Dr. Gawande. I'm the senior surgical resident down here. How are you doing?"

"You're from surgery?" she said, with a look that was part puzzlement and part alarm. I tried to reassure her. The emergency physician was "only being cautious," I said, and having me see her to make sure it was nothing more than a cellulitis. All I wanted to do was ask a few questions and look at her leg. Could she tell me what had been going on? For a moment she said nothing, still trying to compute what to think about all this. Then she let out a sigh and told me the story.

That weekend she had gone back home to Hartford, Connecticut, to attend a wedding. (She had moved to Boston with some girl-friends the year before, after graduating from Ithaca College, and landed work planning conferences for a downtown law firm.) The wedding had been grand and she had kicked off her shoes and danced the whole night. The morning after, however, she woke up with her left foot feeling sore. She had a week-old blister on the top of her foot from some cruddy sandals she had worn, and now the skin surrounding the blister was red and puffy. She didn't think too much of this at first. When she showed her foot to her father, he said he thought it looked like a bee sting or maybe like she'd gotten stepped on dancing the night before. By late that afternoon, however, riding back to Boston with her boyfriend, "my foot really began killing me," she said. The redness spread, and during the night she got chills and sweats and a fever of one hundred and three degrees. She took ibuprofen every few hours, which got her temperature down but did nothing for the mounting pain. By morning, the redness reached halfway up her calf, and her foot had swelled to the point that she could barely fit it into a sneaker.

Eleanor hobbled in on her roommate's shoulder to see her internist that afternoon and was diagnosed with a cellulitis. Cellulitis is your garden-variety skin infection, the result of perfectly ordinary bacteria in the environment getting past the barrier of your skin (through a cut, a puncture wound, a blister, whatever) and proliferating within it. Your skin becomes red, hot, swollen, and painful; you feel sick; fevers are common; and the infection can spread along your skin readily—precisely the findings Eleanor had. The doctor got an X ray to make sure the bone underneath was not infected. Satisfied that it was not, she gave Eleanor a dose of intravenous antibiotics in the office, a tetanus shot, and a prescription for a week's worth of antibiotic pills. This was generally sufficient treatment for a cellulitis, but not always, the doctor warned. Using an indelible black marker, she traced the border of the redness on Eleanor's calf. If the redness should extend beyond this line, the doctor instructed, she should call. And, regardless, she should return the next day for the infection to be checked.

The next morning, Eleanor said—this morning—she woke up with the rash beyond the black line, a portion stretching to her thigh, and the pain worse than ever. She phoned the doctor, who told her to go to the emergency room. She'd need to be admitted to the hospital for a full course of intravenous antibiotic treatment, the doctor explained.

I asked Eleanor if she had had any pus or drainage from her leg. No. Any ulcers open up in her skin? No. A foul smell or blackening of her skin? No. Any more fevers? Not since two days ago. I let the data roll around in my head. Everything was going for a cellulitis. But something was pricking at me, making me alert.

I asked Eleanor if I could see the rash. She pulled back the sheet. The right leg looked fine. The left leg was red—a beefy, uniform, angry red—from her forefoot, across her ankle, up her calf, past the black ink line from the day before, to her knee, with a further tongue of crimson extending to the inside of her thigh. The border was sharp. The skin was hot and tender to the touch. The blister on the top of her foot was tiny. Around it the skin was slightly bruised. Her toes were uninvolved, and she wiggled them for me without difficulty. She had a harder time moving the foot itself—it was thick with edema up through the ankle. She had normal sensation and pulses throughout her leg. She had no ulcers or pus.

Objectively, the rash had the exact appearance of a cellulitis, something antibiotics would take care of. But another possibility lodged in my mind now, one that scared the hell out of me. It was not for logical reasons, though. And I knew this perfectly well.

Decisions in medicine are supposed to rest on concrete observations and hard evidence. But just a few weeks before, I had taken care of a patient I could not erase from my mind. He was a healthy fifty-eight-year-old man who had had three or four days of increasing pain in the left side of his chest, under his arm, where he had an abrasion from a fall. (For reasons of confidentiality, some identifying details have been changed.) He went to a community hospital near his home to get it checked out. He was found to have a small and very ordinary skin rash on his chest and was sent home with antibiotic pills for cellulitis. That night the rash spread eight inches. The following morning he spiked a fever of one hundred and two degrees. By the time he returned to the emergency room, the skin involved had become numb and widely blistered. Shortly after, he went into shock. He was transferred to my hospital and we quickly took him to the OR.

He didn't have a cellulitis but instead an extremely rare and horrendously lethal type of infection known as necrotizing fasciitis (fa-shee-EYE-tiss). The tabloids have called it a disease of "flesh-eating bacteria" and the term is not an exaggeration. Opening the skin, we found a massive infection, far worse than what appeared from the outside. All the muscles of the left side of his chest, going around to his back, up to his shoulder, and down to his abdomen, had turned gray and soft and foul with invading bacteria and had to be removed. That first day in the OR, we had had to take even the muscles between his ribs, a procedure called a birdcage thoracotomy. The next day we had to remove his arm. For a while, we actually thought we had saved him. His fevers went away and the plastic surgeons reconstructed his chest and abdominal wall with transfers of muscle and sheets of Gortex. One by one, however, his kidneys, lungs, liver, and heart went into failure, and then he died. It was among the most awful cases I have ever been involved in.

What we know about necrotizing fasciitis is this: it is highly aggressive and rapidly invasive. It kills up to 70 percent of the people who get it. No known antibiotic will stop it. The most common bacterium involved is group A *Streptococcus* (and, in fact, the final cultures from our patient's tissue grew out precisely this). It is an organism that usually causes little more than a strep throat, but in certain strains it has evolved the ability to do far worse. No one knows where these strains come from. As with a cellulitis, they are understood to enter through breaks in the skin. The break can be as large as a surgical incision or as slight as an abrasion. (People have been documented to have gotten the disease from a rug burn, a bug bite, a friendly punch in the arm, a paper cut, a blood draw, a toothpick injury, and chicken pox lesions. In many the entry point is never found at all.) Unlike with a cellulitis, the bacteria invade not only skin but also deep underneath, advancing rapidly along the outer sheaths of muscle (the fascia) and consuming whatever soft tissue (fat, muscle, nerves, connective tissue) they find. Survival is possible only with early and radical excisional surgery, often requiring amputation. To succeed, however, it must be done early. By the time signs of deep invasion are obvious—such as shock, loss of sensation, widespread blistering of the skin—the person is usually unsalvageable.

Standing at Eleanor's bedside, bent over examining her leg, I felt a little foolish considering the diagnosis—it was a bit like thinking the ebola virus had walked into the ER. True, in the early stages, a necrotizing fasciitis can look just like a cellulitis, presenting with the same redness, swelling, fever, and high white blood cell count. But there is an old saying taught in medical school: if you hear hoofbeats in Texas, think horses not zebras. Only about a thousand cases of necrotizing fasciitis occur in the entire United States each year, mainly in the elderly and chronically ill—and well over *three million* cases of cellulitis. What's more, Eleanor's fever had gone away; she didn't look unusually ill; and I knew I was letting myself be swayed by a single, recent, anecdotal case. If there were a simple test to tell the two diagnoses apart, that would have been one thing. But there is none. The only way is to go to the operating room, open the skin, and look—not something you want to propose arbitrarily.

Yet here I was. I couldn't help it. I was thinking it.

I pulled the sheets back over Eleanor's legs. "I'll be back in a minute," I said. I went to a phone well out of her earshot and paged Thaddeus Studdert, the general surgeon on call. He called back from the OR and I quickly outlined the facts of the case. I told him the rash was probably just a cellulitis. But then I told him there was still one other possibility that I couldn't get out of my head: a necrotizing fasciitis.

The line went silent for a beat.

"Are you serious?" he said.

"Yes," I said, trying not to hedge. I heard an epithet muttered. He'd be right up, he said.

As I hung up the phone, Eleanor's father, a brown-and-gray-haired man in his fifties, came around with a sandwich and soda for her. He had been with her all day, having driven up from Hartford, but when I was seeing her, it turned out, he had been gone getting her lunch. Catching sight of the food, I jumped to tell him not to let her eat or drink "just yet" and with that the cat began crawling out of the bag. It was not the best way to introduce myself. He was immediately taken aback, recognizing that an empty stomach is what we require for patients going to surgery. I tried to smooth matters over, saying that holding off was merely "routine procedure" until we had finished our evaluation. Nonetheless, Eleanor and her father looked on with new dread when Studdert arrived in his scrubs and operating hat to see her.

He had her tell her story again and then uncovered her leg to examine it. He didn't seem too impressed. Talking by ourselves, he told me that the rash looked to him only "like a bad cellulitis." But could he say for sure that it was not necrotizing fasciitis? He could not. It is a reality of medicine that choosing to *not* do something—to not order a test, to not give an antibiotic, to not take a patient to the operating room—is far harder than choosing to do it. Once a possibility has been put in your mind—especially one as horrible as necrotizing fasciitis—the possibility does not easily go away.

Studdert sat down on the edge of her bed. He told Eleanor and her dad that her story, symptoms, and exam all fit with cellulitis and that that was what she most likely had. But there was another, very rare possibility, and, in a quiet and gentle voice, he went on to explain the unquiet and ungentle effects of necrotizing fasciitis. He told them of the "flesh-eating bacteria," the troublingly high death rate, the resistance to treatment by antibiotics alone. "I think it is unlikely you have it," he told Eleanor. "I'd put the chances"—he was guessing here—"at well under five percent." But, he went on, "without a biopsy, we cannot rule it out." He paused for a moment to let her and her father absorb this. Then he started to explain what the procedure involved—how he would take an inch or so of skin plus underlying tissue from the top of her foot, and perhaps from higher up on her leg, and then have a pathologist immediately look at the samples under the microscope.

Eleanor went rigid. "This is crazy," she said. "This doesn't make any sense." She looked frantic, like someone drowning. "Why don't we just wait and see how the antibiotics go?" Studdert explained that this was a disease that you cannot sit on, that you had to catch it early to have any chance of treating it. Eleanor just shook her head and looked down at her covers.

Studdert and I both turned to her father to see what he might have to say. He had been silent to this point, standing beside her, his brow knitted, hands gripped behind him, tense, like a man trying to stay upright on a pitching boat. He asked about specifics—how long a biopsy would take (fifteen minutes), what the risks were (a deep wound infection was the biggest one, ironically), whether the scars go away (no), when it would be done if it were done (within the hour). More gingerly, he asked what would happen if the biopsy were positive for the disease. Studdert repeated that he thought the chances were less than 5 percent. But if she had it, he said, we'd have to "remove all the infected tissue." He hesitated before going on. "This can mean an amputation," he said. Eleanor began to cry. "I don't want to do this, Dad." Mr. Bratton swallowed hard, his gaze fixed somewhere miles beyond us.

In recent years, we in medicine have discovered how discouragingly often we turn out to do wrong by patients. For one thing, where the knowledge of what the right thing to do exists, we still too frequently fail to do it. Plain old mistakes of execution are not uncommon, and we have only begun to recognize the systemic frailties, technological faults, and human inadequacies that cause them, let alone how to reduce them. Furthermore, important knowledge has simply not made its way far enough into practice. Among patients recognized as having heart attacks, for example, it is now known that an aspirin alone will save lives and that even more can be saved with the immediate use of a thrombolytic—a clot-dissolving drug. A quarter of those who should get an aspirin do not, however; and half who should get a thrombolytic do not. Overall, physician compliance with various evidence-based guidelines ranges from over 80 percent of patients in some parts of the country to less than 20 percent in others. Much of medicine still lacks the basic organization and commitment to make sure we do what we know to do.

But spend almost any amount of time with doctors and patients, and you will find that the larger, starker, and more painful difficulty is the still abundant uncertainty that exists over what should be done in many situations. The gray zones in medicine are considerable, and every day we confront situations like Eleanor's—ones in which clear scientific evidence of what to do is missing and yet choices must be made. Exactly which patients with pneumonia, for example, should be hospitalized and which ones sent home? Which back pains treated by surgery and which by conservative measures alone? Which patients with a rash taken to surgery and which just observed on antibiotics? For many cases, the answers can be obvious. But for many others, we simply do not know. Expert panels asked to review actual medical decisions have found that in a quarter of hysterectomy cases, a third of operations to put tubes in children's ears, and a third of pacemaker insertions (to pick just three examples), the science did not exist to say whether the procedures would help those particular patients or not.

In the absence of algorithms and evidence about what to do, you learn in medicine to make decisions by feel. You count on experience and judgment. And it is hard not to be troubled by this.

A couple weeks before seeing Eleanor, I had seen an arthritic and rather elderly woman (she was born before Woodrow Wilson was president) who had come in complaining of a searing abdominal pain that radiated into her back. I learned that she had recently been found to have an aortic aneurysm in her abdomen and instantly my alarm bells went off. Examining her gingerly, I could feel the aneurysm, a throbbing and tender mass just deep to her abdominal muscles. She was stable, but it was on the verge of rupturing, I was convinced. The vascular surgeon I called in agreed. We told the woman that immediate surgery was the only option to save her. We warned her, however, that it was a big surgery, with a long recovery in intensive care and probably in a nursing home afterward (she still lived independently), a high risk that her kidneys would not make it, and a minimum 10 to 20 percent chance of death. She did not know what to do. We left her with her family to think on the decision, and then I returned fifteen minutes later. She said she would not go ahead with surgery. She just wanted to go home. She had lived a long life, she said. Her health had long been failing. She had drawn up her will and was already measuring her remaining days in coffee spoons. Her family was devastated, but she was steady-voiced and constant. I wrote out a pain medication prescription for her son to fill for her, and half an hour later she left, understanding full well that she would die. I kept her son's number and, when a couple weeks had passed, called him at home to hear how he had weathered the aftermath. His mother, however, answered the telephone herself. I stammered a hello and asked how she was doing. She was doing, well, she said, thank you. A year later, I learned, she was still alive and living on her own.

Three decades of neuropsychology research have shown us numerous ways in which human judgment, like memory and hearing, is prone to systematic mistakes. The mind overestimates vivid dangers, falls into ruts, and manages multiple pieces of data poorly. It is swayed unduly by desire and emotion and even the time of day. It is affected by the order in which information is presented and how problems are framed. And if we doctors believed that, with all our training and experience, we escape such fallibilities, the notion was dashed when researchers put us under the microscope.

A variety of studies have shown physician judgment to have these same distortions. One, for example, from the Medical College of Virginia, found that doctors ordering blood cultures for patients with fever overestimated the probability of infection by four- to tenfold. Moreover, the highest overestimates came from the doctors who had recently seen *other* patients with a blood infection. Another, from the University of Wisconsin, found evidence of a Lake Wobegon effect ("Lake Wobegon: where the women are strong, the men are good-looking, and all the children are above average"): the vast majority of surgeons believed the mortality rate for their own patients to be lower than the average. A study from Ohio University and Case Western Reserve Medical School examined not just the accuracy but also the confidence of physicians' judgments—and found no connection between them. Doctors with high confidence in a judgment they made proved no more accurate than doctors with low confidence.

David Eddy, a physician and expert on clinical decision making, reviewed the evidence in an unflinching series of articles published over a decade ago in the *Journal of the American Medical Association*. And his conclusion was damning. "The plain fact is," he wrote, "that many decisions made by physicians appear to be arbitrary—highly variable, with no obvious explanation. The very disturbing implication is that this arbitrariness represents, for at least some patients, suboptimal or even harmful care."

But in the face of uncertainty, what other than judgment does a physician have—or a patient have, for that matter? Months after seeing Eleanor that spring afternoon, I spoke with her father about the events that had unfolded.

"It felt like it was five minutes from having a swollen foot to being told that she could possibly be losing her life," Mr. Bratton said.

A chef who had owned his own delicatessen for seventeen years and now taught at a culinary arts school in Hartford, he knew no one in Boston. He knew our hospital was affiliated with Harvard, but he knew enough to realize that this did not necessarily mean we were anything special. I was just the resident on duty that day; Studdert was likewise just the surgeon on call. Eleanor had left things to her father now, and he tried to take stock. Some clues were encouraging. Studdert's being in scrubs and an operating hat, having just come from the OR, seemed to suggest experience and know-how. Indeed, it turned out he had seen a number of patients with necrotizing fasciitis before. He was also self-assured, without being bullying, and took time to explain everything. But Bratton was shocked at how young he appeared. (Studdert was, in fact, just thirty-five.)

"This is my daughter we are talking about," Bratton remembered thinking at the time. "Isn't there anybody better than you?" Then he knew what to do. He turned to Studdert and me and spoke softly.

"I'd like another opinion," was what he said.

We agreed to the request, and it did not upset us. We were not oblivious to the conundrums here. Eleanor's fever had gone away; she didn't look unusually ill; and likely the biggest reason I had thought of flesh-eating bacteria was that terrible case I had seen a few weeks before. Studdert had put a numeric estimate on the chances of the disease—"well under five percent" he had said—but we both knew it was a stab in the dark (a measure of probability and confidence, but how good is that?) and a vague one at that (how *much* less than 5 percent?). Hearing what someone else might think seemed useful, we both thought.

But, for the Brattons, I had to wonder how useful it would be. If opinions disagreed, then what? And if they did not, wouldn't the same fallibilities and questions remain? Furthermore, the Brattons did not know anyone to call and had to ask if *we* had any ideas.

We suggested calling David Segal, a plastic surgeon on staff who like Studdert had seen such cases before. They agreed. I called Segal and filled him in. He came down within minutes. In the end what he gave Eleanor and her father was mainly confidence, from what I could see.

Segal is a rumpled and complexly haired man, with pen stains on his white coat and glasses that seem too large for his face. He is the only plastic surgeon I know who looks like he has a Ph.D. from M.I.T. (which, as it happens, he does). But he seemed, as Bratton later put it, "not young." And he did not disagree with what Studdert had said. He listened to Eleanor's story and looked carefully at her leg and then said that he too would be surprised if she turned out to have the bacteria. But he agreed that it could not be ruled out. So what else was there but to biopsy?

Eleanor and her dad now agreed to go ahead. "Let's get it over with," she said. But then I brought her the surgical consent form to sign. On it, I had written not only that the procedure was a "biopsy of the left lower extremity" but also that the risks included a "possible need for amputation." She cried out when she saw the words. It took her several minutes alone with her father before she could sign. We had her in the operating room almost immediately after. A nurse brought her father to the family waiting area. He tracked her mother down by cell phone. Then he sat and bowed his head, and made some prayers for his child.

There is, in fact, another approach to decision making, one advocated by a small and struggling coterie in medicine. The strategy, long used in business and the military, is called decision analysis, and the principles are straightforward. On a piece of paper (or a computer), you lay out all your options, and all the possible outcomes of those options, in a decision tree. You make a numeric estimate of the probability of each outcome, using hard data when you have it and a rough prediction when you don't. You weigh each outcome according to its relative desirability (or "utility") to the patient. Then you multiply out the numbers for each option and choose the one with the highest calculated "expected utility." The goal is to use explicit, logical, statistical thinking instead of just your gut. The decision to recommend annual mammograms for all women over age fifty was made this way and so was the U.S. decision to bail out Mexico when its economy tanked. Why not, the advocates ask, individual patient decisions?

Recently, I tried "treeing out" (as the decision buffs put it) the choice Eleanor faced. The options were simple: to biopsy or not biopsy. The outcomes quickly got complicated, however. There was: not being biopsied and doing fine; not being biopsied, getting diagnosed late, going through surgery, and surviving anyway; not being biopsied and dying; being biopsied and getting only a scar; being biopsied and getting a scar plus bleeding from it; being biopsied, having the disease and an amputation, but dying anyway; and so on. When all the possibilities and consequences were penciled out, my decision tree looked more like a bush. Assigning the probabilities for each potential twist of fate seemed iffy. I found what data I could from the medical literature and then had to extrapolate a good deal. And determining the relative desirability of the outcomes seemed impossible, even after talking to Eleanor about them. Is dying a hundred times worse than doing fine, a thousand times worse, a million? Where does a scar with bleeding fit in? Nonetheless, these are the crucial considerations, the decision experts argue, and when we decide by instinct, they say, we are only papering this reality over.

Producing a formal analysis in any practical time frame proved to be out of the question, though. It took a couple of days—not the minutes that we had actually had—and a lot of back and forths with two decision experts. But it did provide an answer. According to the final decision tree, we should *not* have gone to the OR for a biopsy. The likelihood of my initial hunch being right was too low, and the likelihood that catching the disease early would make no difference anyway was too high. Biopsy could not be justified, the logic said.

I don't know what we would have made of this information at the time. We didn't have the decision tree, however. And we went to the OR.

The anesthesiologist put Eleanor to sleep. A nurse then painted her leg with antiseptic, from her toes up to her hip. With a small knife, Studdert cut out an inch-long ellipse of skin and tissue from the top of her foot, where the blister was, down to her tendon. The specimen was plopped into a jar of sterile saline and rushed to the pathologist to look at. We then took a second specimen—going deeper now, down into muscle—from the center of the redness in her calf, and this was sent on as well.

At first glance beneath her skin, there was nothing apparent to alarm us. The fat layer was yellow, as it is supposed to be, and the muscle was a healthy glistening red and bled appropriately. When we probed with the tip of a clamp inside the calf incision, however, it slid unnaturally easily along the muscle, as if bacteria had paved a path. This is not a definitive finding, but enough of one that Studdert let out a sudden, disbelieving, "Oh shit." He pulled off his gloves and gown to go see what the pathologist had found, and I followed right behind him, leaving Eleanor asleep in the OR to be watched over by another resident and the anesthesiologist.

An emergent pathology examination is called a frozen section, and the frozen section room was just a few doors down the hallway. The room was small, the size of a kitchen. In the middle of it stood a waist-high laboratory table with a black slate countertop and a canister of liquid nitrogen in which the pathologist had quick-frozen the tissue samples. Along a wall was the microtome that he had used to slice micron-thin sections of the tissue to put on glass slides. We walked in just as he finished preparing the slides. He took them to a microscope and began scanning each one methodically, initially under low power magnification and then under high power. We hovered, no doubt annoyingly, awaiting the diagnosis. Minutes passed in silence.

"I don't know," the pathologist muttered, still staring through the eyepieces. The features he saw were "consistent with necrotizing fasciitis," he said, but he wasn't sure he could clinch the diagnosis. He said he would have to call in a dermatopathologist, a pathologist who specializes in looking at skin and soft tissue. It took twenty minutes before the specialist arrived and another five before he could make his call, our frustration growing. "She's got it," he finally announced grimly. He had detected some tiny patches where the deep tissue had begun to die. No cellulitis could do that, he said.

Studdert went to see Eleanor's father. When he walked into the crowded family waiting area, Bratton caught the expression on his face and began yelling, "Don't look at me like that! *Don't look at me like that!*" Studdert took him to a private side room, closed the door behind them, and told him that she appeared to have the disease. He would have to move fast, he said. He was not sure he could save her leg and he was not sure if he could save her life. He would need to open her leg up, see how bad things were, and then go from there. Bratton was overcome, crying and struggling to get out words. Studdert's own eyes were wet. Bratton said to "do what you have to do." Studdert nodded and left. Bratton then called his wife. He told her the news and then gave her a moment to reply. "I will never forget what I heard on the other end of the line," he later said. "Something, some sound, I cannot and will never be able to describe."

Decisions compound themselves, in medicine like in anything else. No sooner have you taken one fork in the road than another and another come upon you. The critical question now was what to do. In the OR, Segal joined Studdert to offer another set of hands. Together they slit open Eleanor's leg, from the base of her toes, across her ankle, to just below her knee, to get a full view of what was going on inside. They pulled the opening wide with retractors.

The disease was grossly visible now. In her foot and most of her calf, the outer, fascial layer of her muscles was gray and dead. A brownish dishwater fluid was seeping out with a faint smell of decay. (Tissue samples and bacterial cultures would later confirm that this was toxic group A *Streptococcus* advancing rapidly up her leg.)

"I thought about a BKA," a below-knee amputation, Studdert says, "even an AKA," an above-knee amputation. No one would have faulted him for doing either. But he found himself balking. "She was such a young girl," he explains. "It may seem harsh to say, but if it was a sixty-year-old man I would've taken the leg without question." This was partly, I think, a purely emotional unwillingness to cut off the limb of a pretty twenty-three-year-old—the kind of sentimentalism that can get you in trouble. But it was also partly instinct again, an instinct that her youth and fundamentally good health might allow him to get by with just removing the most infested tissue (a "debridement") and washing out her foot and leg. Was this a good risk to take, with one of the deadliest bacteria known to man loose in her leg? Who knows? But take it he did.

For two hours, using scissors and electrocautery, he and Segal cut and stripped off the necrotic outer layers of her muscle, starting from the webbing of her toes, going up to the tendons of her calf.

They took out tissue going three-quarters of the way around. Her skin hung from her leg like open coat flaps. Higher up, inside the thigh, they reached fascia that looked pink-white and fresh, very much alive. They poured two liters of sterile saline through the leg, trying to wash out as much of the bacteria as possible.

At the end, Eleanor seemed to be holding steady. Her blood pressure remained normal. Her temperature was ninety-nine degrees. Her oxygen levels were fine. And the worst-looking tissue had been removed from her leg.

But her heart rate was running a bit too fast, one hundred and twenty beats a minute, a sign that the bacteria had provoked a systemic reaction. She was requiring large amounts of intravenous fluid. Her foot looked dead. And her skin was still burning red with infection.

Studdert stood firm with his decision not to take more, but you could see he was uneasy about it. He and Segal conferred and thought of one other thing they could try, an experimental therapy called hyperbaric oxygen. It involved putting Eleanor in one of those pressure chambers they put divers in when they get the bends—a perhaps kooky-sounding notion but not a ludicrous one. Immune cells require oxygen to kill bacteria effectively and putting a person under double or higher atmospheric pressure for a few hours a day increases the oxygen concentration in tissue tremendously. Segal had been impressed by results he had gotten using the therapy in a couple of burn patients with deep wound infections. True, studies had not proven that it would work against necrotizing fasciitis. But suppose it could? Everyone latched onto the treatment immediately. At least it made us feel as if we were doing something about all the infection we were leaving behind.

We did not have a chamber at our hospital, but a hospital across town did. Someone got on the phone and within a few minutes we had a plan for ambulancing Eleanor over with one of our nurses for two hours under 2.5 atmospheres of pressurized oxygen. We left her wound open to drain, laid wet gauze inside it to keep the tissues from desiccating, and wrapped her leg in white bandages. Before sending her over, we wheeled her from the OR to intensive care, where we could make sure she would be stable enough for the trip.

It was eight o'clock at night now. Eleanor woke up nauseated and in pain. But she was sharp-witted enough to surmise from the crowd of nurses and doctors around her that something was wrong.

"Oh God, my leg."

She reached down to find it, and for a few panicked moments she wasn't sure she could. Slowly, she convinced herself that she could see it, touch it, feel it, move it. Studdert put his hand on her arm. He explained what he had found, what he had done, and what more there would be to do. She took the information with more grit and fight than I knew she had. Her whole family had now arrived to be with her, and looked as though an SUV had hit them. But Eleanor pulled the sheet back over her leg, took in the monitors flashing their green and orange lights and the IV lines running into her arms, and said, simply, "OK."

The hyperbaric chamber that night was, as she describes it, "like a glass coffin." She lay inside it on a narrow mattress with nowhere to put her arms except straight down or folded across her chest, a panel of thick plexiglass a foot from her face, and an overhead hatch sealed tight with turns of a heavy wheel. As the pressure increased, her ears kept popping, as if she were diving down into a deep ocean. Once the pressure reached a certain point, she would be stuck, the doctors had cautioned. Even if she should start throwing up, they could not get to her, for the pressure could only be released slowly or it would give her the bends and kill her. "One person had a seizure inside," she remembered them telling her. "It took them twenty minutes to get to him." Lying there enclosed, more ill than she'd ever imagined one could be, she felt far away and almost totally alone. It's just me and the bacteria in here, she thought to herself.

The next morning, we took her back to the operating room, to see if the bacteria had spread. They had. The skin over most of her foot and front of her calf was gangrenous and black and had to be cut off. The edges of fascia we had left behind were dead and had to be excised as well. But her muscle was still viable, including in her foot. And the bacteria had not killed anything up in her thigh. She had no further fevers. Her heart rate had normalized. We repacked her wound with wet gauze and sent her back for more hyperbaric oxygen—two hours twice a day.

We ended up operating on her leg four times in four days. At each operation, we had to take a little more tissue, but each time it was less and less. At the third operation, we found the redness of her skin had finally begun to recede. At the fourth operation, the redness was gone and we could see the pink mossy beginnings of new tissue in the maw of her wound. Only then was Studdert confident that not only had Eleanor survived, but her foot and leg had, too.

It is because intuition sometimes succeeds that we don't know what to do with it. Such successes are not quite the result of logical thinking. But they are not the result of mere luck, either.

Gary Klein, a cognitive psychologist who has spent his career observing people who deal routinely with uncertainty, tells the story of a fire commander he once studied. The lieutenant and his team had pulled up to fight an ordinary-seeming fire in a one-story home. He led the hose crew in through the front and encountered the fire in the back kitchen area. They tried dousing it with water. But the flames came right back at them. They tried spraying the fire again but, once more, found little effect. The team retreated a couple of steps to plan another line of attack. Then suddenly, to the bafflement of his men, the lieutenant ordered them out of the building immediately. Something—he didn't know what—didn't feel right. And as soon as they exited, the floor they'd been standing on collapsed. The seat of the fire turned out to be in the basement, not the back. Had they stayed just a few seconds longer, they would have plunged into the fire themselves.

Human beings have an ability to simply recognize the right thing to do sometimes. Judgment, Klein points out, is rarely a calculated weighing of all options, which we are not good at anyway, but instead an unconscious form of pattern recognition. Reviewing the events afterward, the commander told Klein that he had not thought once about the different possibilities in that house. He still had no idea what made him get his crew out of there. The fire had been difficult, but not to a degree that had ever made him flee before. The only explanations seemed either luck or ESP. But questioning him closely about the details of the scene, Klein identified two clues the lieutenant had taken in without even realizing it at the time. The living room had been *warm*—warmer than he was used to for a contained fire in the back of a house. And the fire was *quiet*, when what he had expected was the fire to be loud and noisy. The lieutenant's mind appeared to have recognized in these and perhaps other clues a dangerous pattern, one that told him to give the all-out order. And, in fact, thinking very hard about the situation could well have undermined the advantage of his intuition.

It is still not apparent to me what the clues were that I was registering when I first saw Eleanor's leg. Likewise, it is not obvious what the signs were that we could get by without an amputation. Yet as arbitrary as our intuitions seem, there must have been some underlying sense to them. What there is no sense to is how anyone could have known that, how anyone can reliably tell when a doctor's intuitions are heading down the right track or spinning wildly off.

For close to thirty years, Dartmouth physician Jack Wennberg has studied decision making in medicine, not up close, the way Gary Klein has, but from about as high up as you can get, looking at American doctors as a whole. And what he has found is a stubborn, overwhelming, and embarrassing degree of inconsistency in what we do. His research has shown, for example, that the likelihood of a doctor sending you for a gallbladder-removal operation varies 270 percent depending on what city you live in; for a hip replacement, 450 percent; for care in an intensive care unit during the last six months of your life, 880 percent. A patient in Santa Barbara, California, is five times more likely to be recommended back surgery for a back pain than one in Bronx, New York. This is, in the main, uncertainty at work, with the varying experience, habits, and intuitions of individual doctors leading to massively different care for people.

How can this be justified? The people who pay for the care certainly do not see how. (That is why insurers bug doctors so constantly to explain our decisions.) Nor might the people who receive it. Eleanor Bratton, without question, would have been treated completely differently depending on where she went, who she saw, or even just when she saw me (before or after that previous necrotizing fasciitis case I'd seen; at 2 A.M. or 2 P.M.; on a quiet or a busy shift). She'd have gotten merely antibiotics at one place, an amputation at another, a debridement at a third. This result seems unconscionable.

People have proposed two strategies for change. One is to shrink the amount of uncertainty in medicine—with research, not on new drugs or operations (which already attracts massive amounts of funding) but on the small but critical everyday decisions that patients and doctors make (which gets shockingly little funding). Everyone understands, though, that a great deal of uncertainty about what to do for people will always remain. (Human disease and lives are too complicated for reality to be otherwise.) So it has also been argued, not unreasonably, that doctors must agree in advance on what should be done in the uncertain situations that arise—spell out our actions ahead of time to take the guesswork out and get some advantage of group decision.

This last goes almost nowhere, though. For it runs counter to everything we doctors believe about ourselves as individuals, about our personal ability to reason out with patients what the best course of action for them is. In all the confusion of different approaches that different doctors take to a given problem, somebody must get it right. And each of us—used to making decisions under uncertainty

every day—remains convinced that that somebody is me. For however many times our judgment may fail us, we each have our
Eleanor Bratton, our great improbable save.

It was a year before I saw Eleanor again. Passing through
Hartford, I called in on her at her family's home, a roomy, spic-and-
span, putty-colored colonial with a galumphy dog and beds of flow-
ers outside. Eleanor had moved back home to recover following her
twelve days in the hospital, intending to stay only temporarily but
instead finding herself nestling in. Returning to a normal life, she
said, was taking some getting used to.

Her leg had taken time to heal, not surprisingly. In her final
operation, done during her last days in the hospital, we had needed
to use a sixty-four-square-inch skin graft, taken from her thigh, to
close the wound. "My little burn," she called the result, rolling up
the leg of her sweatpants to show me.

It wasn't anything you'd call pretty, but the wound looked
remarkably good to my eye. In final form, it was about as broad as
my hand and ran from beneath her knee to her toes. Inevitably, the
skin color was slightly off, and the wound edges were heaped up.
The graft also made her foot and ankle seem wide and bulky. But
the wound had no open areas, as there sometimes can be. And the
grafted skin was soft and pliant, not at all tight or hard or contracted.
Her thigh where the graft had been taken was a bright, cherry red,
but still fading gradually.

Recovering the full use of her leg had been a struggle for her. At
first, coming home, she found she could not stand, her muscles were
so weak and sore. Her leg would collapse right under her. Then,
when she'd built the strength back, she found she still could not
walk. Nerve damage had given her a severe foot drop. She saw
Dr. Studdert and he cautioned her that this was something she
might always have. With several months of intense physical therapy,
however, she trained herself to walk heel-toe again. By the time of

my visit, she was actually jogging. She'd also started back working, taking a job as an assistant at one of the big insurance company headquarters in Hartford.

A year on, Eleanor remained haunted by what happened to her. She still had no idea where the bacteria came from. Perhaps the foot soak and pedicure she had gotten at a small hair-and-nail shop the day before that wedding. Perhaps the grass, outside the wedding reception hall, that she'd danced barefoot through with a conga line. Perhaps somewhere in her own house. Any time she got a cut or a fever, she was stricken with mortal fear. She would not go swimming. She would not immerse herself in a bath. She would not even let the water in the shower cover her feet. Her family was planning a vacation to Florida soon, but the idea of traveling so far from her doctors frightened her.

The odds—the seeming randomness—were what disturbed her most. "First, they say the odds of you getting this are nothing—one in two hundred fifty thousand," she said. "But then I got it. Then they say the odds of my beating it are very low. And I beat those odds." Now, when she asked us doctors if she could get the flesh-eating bacteria again, we told her, once more, the odds are improbably low, one in two hundred fifty thousand, just like before.

"I have trouble when I hear something like that. That means nothing to me," she said. She was sitting on her living room sofa as we talked, her hands folded in her lap, the sun rippling through a bay window behind her. "I don't trust that I won't get it again. I don't trust that I won't get anything else that's strange or we've never heard of, or that anyone we know isn't going to get such a thing."

The possibilities and probabilities are all we have to work with in medicine, though. What we are drawn to in this imperfect science, what we in fact covet in our way, is the alterable moment—the fragile but crystalline opportunity for one's know-how, ability, or just gut instinct to change the course of another's life for the better. In the actual situations that present themselves, however—a despondent woman arrives to see you about a newly diagnosed cancer, a victim bleeding from a terrible injury is brought pale and short of breath from the scene, a fellow physician asks for your opinion about a twenty-three-year-old with a red leg—we can never be sure whether we have such a moment or not. Even less clear is whether the actions we choose will prove either wise or helpful. That our efforts succeed at all is still sometimes a shock to me. But they do. Not always, but often enough.

My conversation with Eleanor wandered for a while. We talked about the friends she'd gotten to see now that she was back in Hartford and her boyfriend, who was something called a "fiber-optic electrician" (though what he actually wanted to do, she said, was "high voltage"), about a movie she had recently gone to, and about how much less squeamish she's discovered herself to be after going through her whole ordeal.

"I feel a lot stronger in some ways," she said. "I feel like there is some kind of purpose, like there has to be some sort of reason that I'm still here.

"I think I am also happier as a person"—able to see things in perspective a bit more. "Sometimes," she went on, "I even feel safer. I came through all right, after all."

That May she did go to Florida. It was windless and hot, and one day, off the eastern coast above Pompano, she put one bare foot in the water and then the other. Finally, against all her fears, Eleanor jumped in and went swimming in the ocean.

The water was beautiful, she says.

Notes on Sources

INTRODUCTION

5 Specialized medical journals are where doctors find much of their information on practical problems. Thus, the specific dangers of the large chest mass in children are detailed in articles such as Azizkhan, R. G., et al., "Life-threatening airway obstruction as a complication to the management of mediastinal masses in children," *Journal of Pediatric Surgery* 20 (1985), pp. 816–22. For the most part, the lessons in articles like these are learned the hard way—from experience. Disaster occurs, and we call that a tragedy. But if someone writes it down, we call it science.

At least two articles explain strategies doctors have found using heart-lung pumps to safely manage patients with tumors like Lee's: one, from a team at the University of Pennsylvania, is in the *ASAIO Journal* 44 (1998), pp. 219–21. Another, from a team in Delhi, India, is in the *Journal of Cardiothoracic and Vascular Anesthesia* 15 (2001), pp. 233–36. Both teams describe finding the strategies not through careful research but the way many breakthroughs are found—through happenstance and necessity.

EDUCATION OF A KNIFE

20 K. Anders Ericsson's book on human performance is *The Road to Excellence* (Mahwah, N.J.: Lawrence Erlbaum Press, 1996).

27 The Great Ormond Street Hospital's landmark report on their learning curve for doing the switch operation is Bull, C., et al., "Scientific, ethical, and logistical considerations in introducing a new operation: a retrospective cohort study from paediatric cardiac surgery," *British Medical Journal* 320 (2000), pp. 1168–73. The British report is quoted in Hasan, A., Pozzi, M., and Hamilton, J. R. L., "New surgical procedures: Can we minimise the learning curve?" *British Medical Journal* 320 (2000), pp. 170–73.

28 The Harvard Business School research is reported in several chapters and papers, including Pisano, G., Bohmer, R., and Edmondson, A., "Organizational Differences in Rates of Learning Evidence from the Adoption of Minimally Invasive Cardiac Surgery," *Management Science* 47 (2001); Bohmer, R., Edmondson, A., and Pisano, G., "Managing new technology in medicine," in Herzlinger, R. E., ed., *Consumer-Driven Health Care* (San Francisco: Jossey-Bass, 2001).

THE COMPUTER AND THE HERNIA FACTORY

37 Edenbrandt's study: Heden, B., Ohlin, H., Rittner, R., and Edenbrandt, L., "Acute myocardial infarction detected in the 12-lead ECG by artificial neural networks," *Circulation* 96 (1997), pp. 1798–1802.

   Baxt, W. G., "Use of an artificial neural network for data analysis in clinical decision-making: the diagnosis of acute coronary occlusion," *Neural Computation* 2 (1990), pp. 480–89.

38 The Shouldice Hospital has published its results widely. One summary is in Bendavid, R., "The Shouldice technique: a canon in hernia repair," *Canadian Journal of Surgery* 40 (1997), pp. 199–205, 207.

43 Meehl, P. E., *Clinical Versus Statistical Prediction: A Theoretical Analysis and Review of the Evidence* (Minneapolis: University of Minnesota Press, 1954).

   Dawes, R. M., Faust, D., and Meehl, P. E., "Clinical versus actuarial judgment," *Science* 243 (1989), pp. 1668–74.

44 A nice tutorial on, and summary of, medical neural networks is in Baxt, W. G., "Application of artificial neural networks to clinical medicine," *Lancet* 346 (1995), pp. 1135–38.

45 Herzlinger, R., *Market-Driven Health Care: Who Wins, Who Loses in the Transformation of America's Largest Service Industry* (Reading, Mass.: Addison-Wesley, 1997).

57 Brennan, T. A., et al., "Incidence of adverse events and negligence in hospitalized patients: results of the Harvard Medical Practice Study I," *New England Journal of Medicine* 324 (1991), pp. 370–76.

Leape, L. L., "Error in medicine," *Journal of the American Medical Association* 272 (1994), pp. 1851–57.

Bates, D. W., et al., "Incidence of adverse drug events and potential adverse drug events," *Journal of the American Medical Association* 274 (1995), pp. 29–34.

Localio, A. R., et al., "Relation between malpractice claims and adverse events due to negligence: results of the Harvard Medical Practice Study III," *New England Journal of Medicine* 325 (1991), pp. 245–51.

63 Reason, J., *Human Error* (Cambridge: Cambridge University Press, 1990).

64 The history of anesthesia's success against error is described in Pierce, E. C., "The 34th Rovenstine Lecture: 40 years behind the mask—safety revisited," *Anesthesiology* 84 (1996), pp. 965–75.

65 Cooper, J. B., et al., "Preventable anesthesia mishaps: a study of human factors," *Anesthesiology* 49 (1978), pp. 399–406.

69 The work of the Northern New England Cardiovascular Disease Study Group has been published in numerous studies, but a summary can be found in Malenka, D. J., and O'Connor, G. T., "The Northern New England Cardiovascular Disease Study Group: a regional collaborative effort for continuous quality improvement in cardiovascular disease," *Joint Commission Journal on Quality Improvement* 24 (1998), pp. 594–600.

70 Brooks, D. C., ed., *Current Review of Laparoscopy*, 2nd ed. (Philadelphia: Current Medicine, 1995).

NINE THOUSAND SURGEONS

75 One can find information about the annual American College of Surgeons convention at www.facs.org.

WHEN GOOD DOCTORS GO BAD

88 The tale of Harold Shipman is described in detail in Eichenwald, K., "True English murder mystery: town's trusted doctor did it," *New York Times*, 13 May 2001, p. A1.

Prosecutors in John Ronald Brown's trial alleged his involvement also included attempting to plug a Los Angeles woman's leaking breast implants with Krazy Glue. He was convicted of second-degree murder in the death of Philip Bondy, whose leg was amputated, and sentenced to fifteen years. For more details see Ciotti, P., "Why did he cut off that man's leg?" *LA Weekly*, 17 December 1999.

For the story of James Burt see Griggs, F., "Breaking Tradition: Doctor Steps in to Stop Maiming 'Surgery of Love,'" *Chicago Tribune*, 25 August 1991, p. 8.

94 For data on substance abuse in doctors see Brook, D., et al., "Substance abuse within the health care community," in Friedman, L. S., et al., eds., *Source Book of Substance Abuse and Addiction* (Philadelphia: Lippincott, 1996).

Two comprehensive sources of information on the occurrence of mental illness in the general population are *Mental Health: A Report of the Surgeon General* (Rockville, Md.: U.S. Department of Health and Human Services, 1999); Kessler, R. C., et al., "Lifetime and 12-month prevalence of DSM-III-R psychiatric disorders in the United States: results from the National Comorbidity Survey," *Archives of General Psychiatry* 51 (1994), pp. 8–19.

The estimate of the percentage of problem physicians comes from Marilynn Rosenthal's review "Promise and reality: professional self-regulation and 'problem' colleagues," in Lens, P., and Van der Wal, G., eds., *Problem Doctors: A Conspiracy of Silence* (Netherlands: IOS Press, 1997), p. 23.

Marilynn Rosenthal's book is *The Incompetent Doctor: Behind Closed Doors* (Philadelphia: Open University Press, 1995).

98 Kent Neff presented the data from his work with problem physicians at the Annenberg Conference on Enhancing Patient Safety and Reducing Errors in Health Care, Rancho Mirage, California, 9 November 1998.

FULL MOON FRIDAY THE THIRTEENTH

111 Scanlon, T. J., et al., "Is Friday the 13th bad for your health?" *British Medical Journal* 307 (1993), pp. 1584–89.

William Feller's study of the Nazi bombing of London was published in his book *An Introduction to Probability Theory* (New York: Wiley, 1968).

On Texas sharpshooting, see Rothman, K. J., *American Journal of Epidemiology* 132 (1990), pp. S6–S13.

112 Buckley, N. A., Whyte, I. M., and Dawson, A. H., "There are days . . . and moons: self-poisoning is not lunacy," *Medical Journal of Australia* 159 (1993), pp. 786–89.

113 Guillon, P., Guillon, D., Pierre, F., and Soutoul, J. H., "Les rythmes saisonnier, hebdomadaire et lunaire des naissances," *Revue Francaise de Gynecologie et d'Obstetrique* 11 (1988), pp. 703–8.

The two best summaries on the moon and human behavior are Martin, S. J., Kelly, I. W., and Saklofske, D. H., "Suicide and lunar cycles: a critical review over twenty-eight years," *Psychological Reports* 71 (1992), pp. 787–95; and Byrnes, G., and Kelly, I. W., "Crisis calls and lunar cycles: a twenty-year review," *Psychological Reports* 71 (1992), pp. 779–85.

THE PAIN PERPLEX

118 There is a wide literature on the puzzle of chronic back pain. Among the texts and studies I found useful were Hadler, N., *Occupational Musculoskeletal Disorders* (Philadelphia: Lippincott Williams and Wilkins, current edition 1999); and Haldeman, S., "Failure of the pathology model to predict back pain," *Spine* 15 (1990), p. 719.

The rather curious findings from back MRIs for people in the general population is from the Cleveland Clinic: Jensen, M. C., et al., "Magnetic Resonance Imaging of the lumbar spine in people without back pain," *New England Journal of Medicine* 331 (1994), pp. 69–73.

119 Hilzenrath, D., "Disability claims rise for doctors," *Washington Post*, 16 February 1998.

120 Descartes's description of pain is found in the *Meditations* (1641).

Henry K. Beecher's studies of battlefield pain were published in two places: "Pain in Men Wounded in Battle," *Bulletin of the U.S. Army Medical Department* 5 (April 1946), pp. 445; and "Relationship of Significance of Wound to Pain Experienced," *Journal of the American Medical Association* 161 (1956), pp. 1609–13.

Ronald Melzack and Patrick Wall's classic paper describing Gate-Control Theory was "Pain Mechanisms: A New Theory," *Science* 150 (1965), pp. 971–79.

122 The various studies described on pain in different populations include Tajet-Foxell, B., and Rose, F. D., "Pain and Pain Tolerance in Professional Ballet Dancers," *British Journal of Sports Medicine* 29 (1995), pp. 31–34; Cogan, R., Spinnato, J. A., "Pain and Discomfort Thresholds in Late Pregnancy," *Pain* 27 (1986), pp. 63–68; Berkley, K. J., "Sex Differences in Pain," *Behavioral and Brain Sciences* 20 (1997), pp. 371–80; Barnes, G. E., "Extraversion and pain," *British Journal of Social and Clinical Psychology* 14 (1975), pp. 303–8; Compton, M. D., "Cold-Pressor Pain Tolerance In Opiate And

Cocaine Abusers: Correlates of Drug Type and Use Status," *Journal of Pain and Symptom Management* 9 (1994), pp. 462–73; and Bandura, A., et al., "Perceived Self-Efficacy and Pain Control: Opioid and Nonopioid Mechanisms," *Journal of Personality and Social Psychology* 53 (1987), pp. 563–71.

123 Frederick Lenz published his two cases in two separate papers: Lenz, F. A., et al., "Stimulation in the human somatosensory thalamus can reproduce both the affective and sensory dimensions of previously experienced pain," *Nature Medicine* 1 (1995), pp. 910–13; and "The sensation of angina can be evoked by stimulation of the human thalamus," *Pain* 59 (1994), pp. 119–25.

125 Melzack's new theory is described in his article "Pain: Present, Past, and Future," *Canadian Journal of Experimental Psychology* 47 (1993), pp. 615–29.

127 Information on new drugs is changing quickly, so I'd recommend looking for the most up-to-date references. But the studies described are from Miljanich, G. P., "Venom peptides as human pharmaceuticals," *Science and Medicine* (September/October 1997), pp. 6–15; and Bannon, A. W., et al., "Broad-Spectrum, Non-Opioid Analgesic Activity by Selective Modulation of Neuronal Nicotinic Acetylcholine Receptors," *Science* 279 (1998), pp. 77–81.

128 The tale of Australia's repetitive stress injury epidemic in the 1980s can be found in Hall, W., and Morrow, L., "Repetition strain injury: an Australian epidemic of upper limb pain," *Social Science and Medicine* 27 (1988), pp. 645–49; Ferguson, D., "'RSI': Putting the epidemic to rest," *Medical Journal of Australia* 147 (1987), p. 213; and Hocking, B., "Epidemiological aspects of 'repetition strain injury' in Telecom Australia," *Medical Journal of Australia* 147 (1987), pp. 218–22.

A QUEASY FEELING

130 For a nice summary of the physiology of vomiting see chapter 1 in Sleisinger, M., ed., *Handbook of Nausea and Vomiting* (New York: Parthenon Publishing Group, 1993).

133 Watcha, M. F., and White, P. F., "Postoperative nausea and vomiting: its etiology, treatment, and prevention," *Anesthesiology* 77 (1992), pp. 162–84.

Griffin, A. M., et al., "On the receiving end: patient perceptions of the side effects of cancer chemotherapy," *Annals of Oncology* 7 (1996), pp. 189–95.

Jewell, D., and Young, G., "Treatments for nausea and vomiting in early pregnancy," *Cochrane Database of Systematic Reviews*, 4 March 2000.

134 Profet, M., "Pregnancy sickness as adaptation: a deterrent to maternal ingestion of teratogens," in Barkow, J. H., Cosmides, L., and Tooby, J., *The Adapted Mind* (Oxford: Oxford University Press, 1992).

135 The classic text on motion sickness is Reason, J. T., and Brand, J. J., *Motion Sickness* (New York: Academic Press, 1975).

A short and useful summary of more recent research on motion sickness, including space sickness, can be found in Oman, C. M., "Motion sickness: a synthesis and evaluation of the sensory conflict theory," *Canadian Journal of Physiology and Pharmacology* 68 (1990), pp. 294–303.

138 Studies described include Fischer-Rasmussen, W., et al., "Ginger treatment of hyperemesis gravidarum," *European Journal of Obstetrics, Gynecology, and Reproductive Biology* 42 (1991), pp. 163–64; O'Brien, B., Relyea, J., and Taerum, T., "Efficacy of P6 acupressure in the treatment of nausea and vomiting during pregnancy," *American Journal of Obstetrics and Gynecology* 174 (1996), pp. 708–15.

A valuable summary reference on care for those with hyperemesis of pregnancy is Nelson-Piercy, C., "Treatment of nausea and vomiting in pregnancy: When should it be treated and what can be safely taken?" *Drug Safety* 19 (1998), pp. 155–64.

140 For a short and balanced summary of marijuana's uses in medicine see Voth, E. A., and Schwartz, R., "Medicinal applications of Delta-9-Tetrahydrocannabinol and marijuana," *Annals of Internal Medicine* 126 (1997), pp. 791–98.

For more on the peculiar entity of rumination syndrome see Malcolm, A., et al., "Rumination syndrome," *Mayo Clinic Proceedings* 72 (1997), pp. 646–52.

The study of Zofran and nausea from Gary Morrow's research group is Roscoe, J. A., et al., "Nausea and vomiting remain a significant clinical problem: trends over time in controlling chemotherapy-induced nausea and vomiting in 1,413 patients treated in community clinical practices," *Journal of Pain & Symptom Management* 20 (2000), pp. 113–21.

An excellent review of the psychology of nausea is Morrow, G. R., "Psychological aspects of nausea and vomiting: anticipation of chemotherapy," in Sleisinger, ed., 1993.

142 The groundbreaking report on a substance P antagonist in nausea was Navari, R. M., et al., "Reduction of cisplatin-induced emesis by a

selective neurokinin-1-receptor antagonist," *New England Journal of Medicine* 340 (1999), pp. 190–95.

　　For a summary of the evidence for benefit from palliative care specialists see Hearn, J., and Higginson, I. J., "Do specialist palliative care teams improve outcomes for cancer patients?: a systematic literature review," *Palliative Medicine* 12 (1998), pp. 317–32.

144　Information about Bendectin is reviewed in Koren, G., Pastuszak, A., and Ito, S., "Drug therapy: drugs in pregnancy," *New England Journal of Medicine* 338 (1998), pp. 1128–37.

　　Cassell, E. G., *The Nature of Suffering and the Goals of Medicine* (New York: Oxford University Press, 1991).

CRIMSON TIDE

149　The Freudian arguments are presented in Karch, F. E., "Blushing," *Psychoanalytic Review* 58 (1971), pp. 37–50.

　　Charles Darwin's essay on blushing is in his book *The Expression of the Emotions in Man and Animals* (1872).

　　Michael Lewis details his demonstration of embarrassment from being stared at in "The self in self-conscious emotions," *Annals of the New York Academy of Sciences* 818 (1997), pp. 119–42.

　　The science and psychology of blushing described here, including Leary and Templeton's study, comes from three sources: Leary, M. R., et al., "Social blushing," *Psychological Bulletin* 112 (1992), pp. 446–60; Miller, R. S., *Embarrassment: Poise and Peril in Everyday Life* (New York: Guilford Press, 1996); and Edelmann, R. J., "Blushing," in Crozier, R., and Alden, L. E., eds., *International Handbook of Social Anxiety* (Chichester: John Wiley & Sons, 2000).

153　The Göteborg surgeons' results with ETS for blushing were published in Drott, C., et al., "Successful treatment of facial blushing by endoscopic transthoracic sympathicotomy," *British Journal of Dermatology* 138 (1998), pp. 639–43. For a more chary view of the surgery, see Drummond, P. D., "A caution about surgical treatment for facial blushing," in *British Journal of Dermatology* 142 (2000), pp. 195–96.

160　The Web site for Christine Drury's organization is www.redmask.org.

THE MAN WHO COULDN'T STOP EATING

162　The statistics on the number of gastric-bypass operations being done comes from Blackburn, G., "Surgery for obesity," *Harvard Health Letter* (2001), no. 884.

169 The National Institutes of Health's depressing findings on the long-term, almost universal failure of dieting is in its publication "Methods for voluntary weight loss and control," *Annals of Internal Medicine* 119 (1993), pp. 764–70.

A fairly comprehensive listing of the various surgical treatments that obese people have been subjected to, and their results, can be found in Kral, J. G., "Surgical treatment of obesity," in Bray, G. A., Bouchard, C., and James, W. P. T., eds., *Handbook of Obesity* (New York: M. Decker, 1998); together with Munro, J. F., et al., "Mechanical treatment for obesity," *Annals of the New York Academy of Sciences* 499 (1987), pp. 305–11.

170 The research on dieting for obese children described is in Epstein, L. H., et al., "Ten-year outcomes of behavioral family-based treatment for childhood obesity," *Health Psychology* 13 (1994), pp. 373–83.

Information on Prader-Willi syndrome comes from Lindgren, A. C., et al., "Eating behavior in Prader-Willi syndrome, normal weight, and obese control groups," *Journal of Pediatrics* 137 (2000), pp. 50–55; and Cassidy, S. B., and Schwartz, S., "Prader-Willi and Angelman syndromes," *Medicine* 77 (1998), pp. 140–51.

The "fat paradox" is explained in Blundell, J. E., "The control of appetite," *Schweizerische* 129 (1999), p. 182.

171 One study demonstrating the "appetizer effect" is Yeomans, M. R., "Rating changes over the course of meals: What do they tell us about motivation to eat?" *Neuroscience and Biobehavioral Reviews* 24 (2000), pp. 249–59.

The French chewing study is published in Bellisle, F., et al., "Chewing and swallowing as indices of the stimulation to eat during meals in humans," *Neuroscience and Biobehavioral Reviews* 24 (2000), pp. 223–28.

171 The study of eating in densely amnesiac people is published in Rozin, P., et al., "What causes humans to begin and end a meal?" *Psychological Science* 9 (1998), pp. 392–96.

173 Information on the long-term failure of just stomach stapling surgery to maintain weight loss is from Blackburn's 2001 article, cited above, and Nightengale, M. L., et al., "Prospective evaluation of vertical banded gastroplasty as the primary operation for morbid obesity," *Mayo Clinic Proceedings* 67 (1992), pp. 304–5.

174 For information on the psychological and social experiences of obesity surgery, see Hsu, L. K. G., et al., "Nonsurgical factors that influence the outcome of bariatric surgery: a review," *Psychosomatic Medicine* 60 (1998), pp. 338–46.

Two excellent summaries of the research on the sustained long-term weight loss from obesity surgery are Kral's 1998 article and Blackburn's 2001 article, both cited above.

181 For data on the high prevalence of morbid obesity, see Kuczmarski, R. J., et al., "Varying body mass index cutoff points to describe overweight prevalence among U.S. adults: NHANES III (1988 to 1994)," *Obesity Research* 5 (1997), pp. 542–48.

FINAL CUT

191 The faltering war on the nonautopsy is recounted in Lundberg, G. D., "Low-tech autopsies in the era of high-tech medicine," *Journal of the American Medical Association* 280 (1998), pp. 1273–74.

192 Information on the history of autopsy comes from two sources: Iserson, K. V., *Death to Dust: What Happens to Dead Bodies* (Tucson, Ariz.: Galen Press, 1994); and King, L. S., and Meehan, M. C., "The history of the autopsy," *American Journal of Pathology* 73 (1973), 514–44.

197 The three recent studies evaluating autopsy are Burton, E. C., Troxclair, D. A., and Newman III, W. P., "Autopsy diagnoses and malignant neoplasms: How often are clinical diagnoses incorrect?" *Journal of the American Medical Association* 280 (1998), pp. 1245–48; Nichols, L., Aronica, P., and Babe, C., "Are autopsies obsolete?" *American Journal of Clinical Pathology* 110 (1996), pp. 210–18; and Zarbo, R. J., Baker, P. B., and Howanitz, P. J., "The autopsy as a performance measurement tool," *Archives of Pathology and Laboratory Medicine* 123 (1999), pp. 191–98.

The review of autopsy studies described is from Hill, R. B., and Anderson, R. E., *The Autopsy: Medical Practice and Public Policy* (Newton, Mass.: Butterworth-Heinemann, 1988), pp. 34–35.

The classic comparison of autopsies over the decades is Goldman, L., et al., "The value of the autopsy in three medical eras," *New England Journal of Medicine* 308 (1983), pp. 1000–5.

198 Gorovitz and MacIntyre's explanation of necessary fallibility is in their article "Toward a theory of medical fallibility," *Journal of Medicine and Philosophy* 1 (1976), pp. 51–71.

201 The disappearance of data on the autopsy is described in Burton, E., "Medical error and outcome measures: Where have all the autopsies gone?" *Medscape General Medicine*, 28 May 2000.

202 The details of the case come mainly from two sources: the affidavit for Marie Noe's arrest and Stephen Fried's disturbing article, "Cradle to Grave," *Philadelphia Magazine*, April 1998.

203 On the reduction of sudden infant deaths associated with the national "Back to Sleep" campaign, see Willingner, M., et al., "Factors associated with the transition to nonprone sleep positions of infants in the United States," *Journal of the American Medical Association* 280 (1998), pp 329–35.

204 A comprehensive source for information on patterns of child abuse is Sedlak, A. J., and Broadhurst, D. D., *The Third National Incident Study of Child Abuse and Neglect* (Washington: U.S. Department of Health and Human Services, 1996).

WHOSE BODY IS IT, ANYWAY?

210 Katz, J., *The Silent World of Doctor and Patient* (New York: Free Press, 1984).

220 The study of what cancer patients prefer is Degner, L. F., and Sloan, J. A., "Decision making during serious illness: What role do patients really want to play?" *Journal of Clinical Epidemiology* 45 (1992), pp. 941–50.

222 Schneider, C. E., *The Practice of Autonomy* (New York: Oxford University Press, 1998).

THE CASE OF THE RED LEG

233 Information on necrotizing fasciitis comes from Chapnick, E. K., and Abter, E. I., "Necrotizing soft-tissue infections," *Infectious Disease Clinics* 10 (1996), pp. 835–55; and Stone, D. R., and Gorbach, S. L., "Necrotizing fasciitis: the changing spectrum," *Infectious Disease in Dermatology* 15 (1997), pp. 213–20. A useful source of information for patients is also the National Necrotizing Fasciitis Foundation Web site, www.nnff.org.

236 For a comprehensive summary of research on the quality of health care (including the heart attack studies described), see Institute of Medicine, *Crossing the Quality Chasm* (Washington, D.C.: National Academy of Sciences Press, 2001).

Naylor, C. D., "Grey zones of clinical practices: some limits to evidence-based medicine," *Lancet* 345 (1995), pp. 840–42.

238 The Medical College of Virginia study: Poses, R. M., and Anthony, M., "Availability, wishful thinking, and physicians' diagnostic judgments

for patients with suspected bacteremia," *Medical Decision Making* 11 (1991), pp. 159–68.

The University of Wisconsin study: Detmer, D. E., Fryback, D. G., and Gassner, K., "Heuristics and biases in medical decision making," *Journal of Medical Education* 53 (1978), pp. 682–83.

The Ohio study: Dawson, N. V., et al., "Hemodynamic assessment in managing the critically ill: Is physician confidence warranted?" *Medical Decision Making* 13 (1993), pp. 258–66.

239 The first installment of David Eddy's startling series on the problems with decision making in medicine is "The challenge," *Journal of the American Medical Association* 263 (1990), pp. 287–90.

247 Gary Klein's magnificent book on his research into intuitive decision making is *Sources of Power* (Cambridge: M.I.T. Press, 1998).

248 One can look up information about the patterns of what doctors in one's own area do relative to doctors in other areas in Jack Wennberg and his research team's publication, *Dartmouth Atlas of Health Care* (Chicago: American Hospital Publishing, Inc., 1999). Their findings are also available online at www.dartmouthatlas.org.

Acknowledgments

Being the child of two doctors, I have been familiar with medicine since I was small. The dinner talk at home was as often about local doctor gossip and cases (the badly asthmatic boy my mom was taking care of, for instance, whose parents were not giving him his medication; my dad's first successfully reversed vasectomy; the guy who'd gone to bed drunk and shot his penis off thinking there was a snake under the covers) as about school and politics. As soon as we were old enough, my sister and I were taught to field phone calls from patients. "Is this an emergency?" we learned to ask. If callers said yes, that was easy. We were to tell them to go to the emergency room. And if they said no, that was easy, too. We were to take a message. Only one time did I get an "I don't know." It was from a man with a rather strained voice calling for my father because he'd "injured himself" while shoveling. I told him to go to the emergency room.

Once in a while, I'd be out with my mom or dad when an emergency page would come through. We'd go to the hospital together, and I'd be put in a chair in the ER hallway to wait. I'd sit watching the sick children crying, the men bleeding into rags, the old ladies breathing funny, and the nurses scurrying everywhere. I got more used to the place than I realized. Years later, as a medical student entering a Boston hospital for my first time, I realized I already knew the smell.

I came to writing, however, only much later and with the help of a lot of people whom I owe a deep debt of gratitude. My friend Jacob Weisberg was the one who first encouraged me to write seriously. He is the chief political correspondent for the Internet magazine *Slate*, and during my second year of surgical residency he pushed me to give a try at some medical writing for his publication. I agreed. He helped me through multiple drafts of that first piece. And then, over the next two years, he and Michael Kinsley, *Slate*'s editor-in-chief, along with my editors Jack Shafer and Jodie Allen, gave me both space and guidance to create what became a regular column on medicine and science. The opportunity changed everything for me. Residency is a grueling experience, and in the midst of all the paperwork and pages and sleep deprivation, you can forget why what you do matters. The writing let me step back and, for a few hours each week, remember.

In my third year of residency, another friend, the *New Yorker* writer Malcolm Gladwell, introduced me to his editor Henry Finder. And for this I consider myself one of the luckiest writers there could be. A mumbling, astonishingly widely read boy genius who at the age of thirty-two was already editor to several of the writers I most admired, Henry took me under his wing. He had the patience and persistence and optimism to pull me through seven complete rewrites of the first article I submitted to *The New Yorker*. He pushed me to think harder than I had ever thought I could. He showed me which of my instincts in writing I could have confidence in and which ones I should not. More than that, he has always believed that I had stories worth telling. Since 1998, *The New Yorker* has engaged me as a staff writer. Many of the chapters in this book originated as articles I published there. In addition, Henry has read and provided invaluable advice on everything written here. This book would not have been possible without him.

There is a third person at *The New Yorker* besides Henry and Malcolm to whom I owe particular thanks: David Remnick. Despite my unpredictable schedule as a resident, and the reality that my patient responsibilities must come first, he has stuck with me. He has built a great and special magazine. And most of all, he has made me feel part of it.

In writing this book, I have found two new kinds of people in my life. One is an agent, which seems like something everyone should have—especially if you can have one like Tina Bennett, who has looked after both me and the book with dedication, unshakable good cheer, and eminently sound judgment in everything (even as she carried and gave birth to a child in the midst of the project). The other is a book editor, which turns out to be a species as different from magazine editors as surgeons are from internists. With an uncommon combination of tenacity and gentleness, Sara Bershtel at Metropolitan Books got me to find the broader frame that caught what it is I write and think about, showed me how a book could be more than I imagined it to be, and somehow kept me going though at times the task seemed overwhelming. I am immensely fortunate to have her. My thanks, too, to her colleague Riva Hochermann, for her careful reading of the manuscript and invaluable suggestions.

Trying to write as a surgical resident is a sensitive and tricky matter, particularly when one is as interested, as I am, in writing about how things go wrong as how things go right. Doctors and hospitals are usually suspicious of efforts to discuss these matters in public. But to my surprise I have found only encouragement where I am. Two people in particular have been instrumental in this. Dr. Troy Brennan, a professor of medicine, law, and almost anything else you can think of, has been a mentor, a sounding board, a collaborator in research, and an unstinting advocate for what I have attempted to do. He even gave me the office space, computer, and phone that let me get this work done.

Dr. Michael Zinner, my hospital's chairman of surgery, has likewise given me his backing and protection. I remember approaching him after I had written my story trying to explain what happens when doctors make mistakes, intending to publish it in *The New Yorker*. I knew it was something I could not publish without permission from him. So I gave him the manuscript and then, a few days later, walked into his office braced for the worst. As it turned out, he didn't love it. How could he? No hospital public relations department in the world would have let an essay like that go out. But he did a remarkable thing: he supported me anyway. The article could easily backfire, he warned me, with the public or with other doctors. But if there was flak he would help me, he promised. And he let me go ahead.

In the end, there never was any flak. Even when my colleagues from work have disagreed with what I've written, they have been constructive and engaged and have held nothing against me. We are all, I've found, in the process of trying to understand how much of what we do is good, how much of it can be better.

To the patients and families who go named and unnamed in this book, I wish to extend a great and special thanks. Some I am fortunate to still keep up with. Others I was never given the chance to know as well as I wish I could have. All of them have taught me more than any could know.

There is just one person, however, who has been involved in all the parts of what is here—the writing, the doctoring, and the struggling to succeed at both: my wife, Kathleen. She's stuck with me through the long hours and turmoil of surgical training and bolstered me when my confidence and resilience have failed me. Then, when I've come home, she's helped me to talk through the ideas I've had for writing and stayed up late with me to help hammer them into words. A magnificent editor herself, she has red-penciled this entire manuscript and, though I've sometimes not wanted to admit it, made everything better. She has also, most critically, kept our sweet and demented children in my life — even bringing them to the hospital to see me when I've missed them and been away for too long. This book exists thanks to her love and dedication. So it is dedicated to her.